THE SICILIAN SECRET DIET PLAN

By

Dr.'s Sandra and Giovanni Campanile

As stated from their opening paragraph, the Campaniles (a psychiatrist and cardiologist duo) state this is not another diet book. Or a weight loss book. It is an engaging history of the massive cultural migrations that swept over the island of Sicily bringing with them the diversity of food and food preparation we know today. This Sicilian cornucopia is, in fact, a direct result of 5,000 years of food enrichment, as nourishment, as a bringer of health and long-sought longevity. The Sicilian island was ready-made for this, positioned perfectly in the Mediterranean Sea amidst the rise and fall of empires and exotic influences from the entire region. The military and culinary crosscurrents from Italy, Greece, the Middle East, Africa, Spain and France swept up on the island's shores bringing a mélange of diversity and nutritional experiments. Over the centuries, these multi-cultural recipes, cooking techniques, plants, and spices distilled into what the Dr.s Campanile cogently argue became the most balanced, salubrious, longevity-inducing palette available for our tables and our bodies today. Not only an engaging read but a fact-filled overview of the intricate interconnection between food and our well being, this book will open a vision far beyond diet, far beyond weight loss, to the essence of wellness itself.

…Rob Cohen….
(Director of 'THE FAST AND THE FURIOUS')

THE
SICILIAN
SECRET
DIET PLAN

**How 5000 years of culinary influence from Italy,
Greece, the Middle East, Africa, Spain and France
has led to the perfect diet for humanity today**

by Giovanni and Sandra Campanile

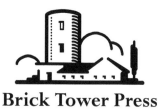

Brick Tower Press
Habent Sua Fata Libelli

Manhanset House
Dering Harbor, New York 11965-0342
bricktower@aol.com
www.BrickTowerPress.com

Copyright © 2021 by Giovanni Campanile, Sandra Cammarata
First Edition
Library of Congress Cataloging in Publication Data
Campanile, Giovanni.
Cammarata, Sandra.

Nutritional advisor:
Francesca Maria Campanile, RN
Nutritionist
Doctoral Candidate, Columbia University

Interior design by Glen M. Edelstein

The Sicilian Secret Diet Plan.
1. COOKING—Regional & Ethnic—Italian. 2. COOKING—Health & Healing—General. 3. HEALTH & FITNESS—Longevity. I. Title.

ISBN: Trade b/w, 978-1-899694-71-6; Trade 4-color, 978-1-899694-96-9; Library, 978-1-899694-97-6
March 2021
The publisher does not offer medical advice. Please consult with your physician if you have any questions.

FROM SANDRA:

To Maria Bonetta-Cammarata who has best expressed her love for her family and friends through the love and respect of the Sicilian cuisine. It is to my mother that I owe all that I know about food. She has taught me how to respect the seasonality of the ingredients, how to understand the timing of cooking to bring out the right flavor, how to trust my eyes, my smell and my taste and most of all she has taught me to be proud of what I serve in my kitchen because food is the best expression of pure love.

FROM GIOVANNI:

To Maria Barbaro-Campanile who has carried and protected her home recipes through her voyage across the Atlantic. It is my mother who has taught me to be proud of the hard work that it takes to protect traditions. She defended her fresh sauces against the quick meals readily available in her adopted country. It is her love that has given me and my four siblings the same respect for the traditions that she worked so hard to preserve.

The two Marias have both unfortunately passed on, however, they are with us both in spirit and in every dish that they have left for us to make for ourselves and the younger generations in our family that are also learning the same traditions.

CONTENTS

INTRODUCTION

THIS IS NOT A DIET BOOK. It is a guide to a lifestyle inspired by the wisdom of our ancestors and the flavor of their food. We are going to take you to a journey to Sicily, walk through her history, experience her passion and taste the simple and nutritious recipes created by her rich volcanic soil, her burning sun and her deep, clear sea waters. We will be sharing with you the scientific data that support the evidence of that wisdom.

Sicily, "umbilicus mundi", (belly button of the world) has been forever the protagonist of the history of humanity and a fierce protectionist of recipes that have been transmitted orally and in writing for many generations and over thousands of years.

My wife Sandra and I are physicians who believe that good nutrition is fundamental to improve the health span and the life span of our patients. Our daughter is a nutritionist, our son is a permaculture farmer and his wife is a physician who also treats her patients with nutrition and lifestyle change.

Sicily is the home of many Centenaries. Centenarians are people that live to be over 100 years old and supercentenarians are those that live beyond 110 years of age. It is our deepest conviction, after caring for many patients and having studied the lifestyle and diets of Sicilian centenaries, that there is a way of eating and living that promotes health that is truly a better and more enjoyable way of experiencing life.

Our mission in writing this book is to present to you the Sicilian lifestyle that has been successfully practiced for three thousand years and has helped Sicilians live long and well. The Sicilian way of eating and living can be easily adopted into anyone's daily routine.

As nutritionally focused physicians we have written this book in order to present a way of eating that we believe is the best version of the Mediterranean diet. This is The Sicilian Secret we want to share with you.

The first rule of good nutrition is that the food has to be delicious, The Sicilian Mediterranean diet is unique because it has been influenced by the many cultures that have invaded and settled in Sicily. These populations of conquerors added their food heritage to the Sicilian cuisine. The Sicilians artfully integrated it into theirs and the result is a diet that is both delicious, interesting and health promoting.

Sandra was born and raised in Sicily and we have been traveling there for over 30 years, observing and studying the lifestyle and diet of the local population. We have met many wonderful people who live simple healthy lives. Sicily has been both cursed and blessed by its poverty and isolation from mainland Italy. Many Italian immigrants to America have come from Sicily because of this extreme poverty. However, because of this isolation, Sicily was passed over to a certain degree by modernity and was able to maintain its traditional ways of life and food culture to a greater degree than other areas of Europe that quickly changed after the industrial revolution.

Many Americans have never learned the basics of healthy eating. The United States is in the middle of a national eating disorder crisis. It is estimated that our poor eating habits cause 700,000 deaths each year because of obesity, heart disease, strokes, diabetes, decreased immunity, and dementia. Americans eat a dismal amount of whole foods like fruits and vegetables and an excessive amount of processed food that contains added salt, sugar and saturated fats. In addition, our consumption of red meats and sugary drinks are excessive. The obesity rate in U.S. children is rising so fast that it is estimated that 60% of today's children will be obese by age 35 if the trend is not reversed. Since obesity is very difficult to turn around at any age, adults need to change and adopt healthy lifestyles for themselves and their children.

Let us become the best ancestors we can be.

A Brief History *of* Sicilian Food

SICILY IS AN ISLAND IN the middle of the Mediterranean Sea and because of its strategic location it was the center of the most important naval routes. As an island, it offered natural vantage points to view and defend from enemies approaching by water. At 10,000 square miles, it is the largest island in the Mediterranean and is blessed with harbors and hills, rich volcanic soil, plentiful fresh water, a temperate climate and long growing seasons. Different cultures and populations have conquered and inhabited the island bringing with them their traditions and leaving behind their culinary histories. Sicily has belonged to many civilizations but it has never been part of any.

Unlike what has happened in many other cultures, in Sicily the new never displaced the old and the new culinary recipes found strengths in the old ones. In the Sicilian culture and history traditions and innovations live in harmony and the past and present walk hand in hand.

The mild climate, the fertile terrain and the abundance of fish have helped to give birth to a cuisine that has successfully integrated multiple cultures. Nature and history have contributed to the heterogeneity and the uniqueness of the Sicilian diet.

Humans arrived in Sicily at the same time that Homo Sapiens appeared as a species, 5 or 6 million years ago through the Africa-Asia-Europe-Sicily migration. The Sikanians inhabited the Island 3000 years ago possibly reaching Sicily from Spain or Ligury. The Siculi arrived in Sicily in 1400 BC from the middle East and the Balkans. The name Siculi means Sickle, they were a population of farmers who later learned the art of navigation to become fishermen in addition to farmers.

Following the Siculi, the Greeks arrived. From then on, a colorful parade followed. Phoenicians (from modern day Syria), Carthaginians from northern Africa, Persians, Romans, Turks, Tunisians, Normans, Swabians (from what is now southwest Germany), French, Spaniards, and the Vikings. They came and conquered leaving behind traces of their languages, architecture, art, and cuisine. They also left behind their genes.

The Sikanians built lava rock mills for their grains and cooked their meats on the grill. We believe that the first dessert that humans consumed might have been made in Sicily with honey and fresh ricotta cheese. A famous dessert the "cuccia" is still made today in some parts of Sicily and is very similar to that very first Sicilian dessert.

In Homer's Odyssey we find the beginning traces of the future importance of Sicilian gastronomic history and through these writings the export of the Sicilian cuisine around the world began. Ulysses discovered pecorino cheese in Polyphemus's cave! Barley was most likely the first cereal cultivated in Sicily. It was toasted and then minced to make a flour that when boiled in water transformed into in a very nutritious food. With the discovery of grains, nutrition improved and it was necessary to eat less to feel satiated. Without the Greeks or the Arabs the Sicilian landscape would probably be very different today. The oranges, lemon trees, grapevines and olive trees that today enthusiastically represent Sicily, were introduced by the populations that conquered and inhabited the island.

The Phoenicians, the Carthaginians and the Greeks have left their traces in the way the modern day Sicilians make their breads and in the way they cure their olives or salt their ricotta.

The Phoenicians promoted the culture of olives, they taught Sicilians how to extract salt from the sea, how to care for livestock, how to keep wine in ceramic containers, the art of apiculture and the fish industry. Their meals were rich in grains and legumes. They ate vegetables raw or cooked, meat was eaten only occasionally and they especially enjoyed rabbit with its lean meat.

Sicilian cuisine was loved by the ancient Greeks. A famous ancient Greek man, named Miteco, from Syracuse, the largest Greek colony in the world which was located on the east coast of Sicily, taught the Greeks the finer points of Sicilian cooking, which he felt to be the best in the world. In reality, Sicilian cuisine was very simple then and consisted of fish, meats (rabbit, goat, sheep) flavored with garlic and aromatic herbs, cooked over an open fire, with raw or cooked vegetables. The wine was locally produced and was already well regarded throughout the Mediterranean basin. Sicilian desserts were famous throughout Italy, Greece, and the Near East. Aristocratic Greek families insisted on having Sicilian cooks, and subsequently when the Romans ruled, wealthy Roman families also made sure that their food was prepared by a Sicilian. Latin writings from the ancient Romans read, "Siculus coquus et Siculus mensa" (Sicilian cooks and Sicilian cuisine). The Sicilian diet had a tremendous impact on the culture and lifestyle of the inhabitants of the Roman Empire.

Sicily was considered the bread basket of the Roman Empire, and produced large quantities of durum wheat which was a basic staple of the diet of Sicily and of the entire Roman Empire. Puls is a dish made from farro grains flavored with salt and herbs, and was an aboriginal food made in Sicily and consumed by the ancient Romans throughout Italy and the Roman Empire. These foods were also part of ancient Roman religious' rituals and festivals. Legumes were grown and prepared by Sicilians, and enjoyed by ancient people throughout the Roman Empire, and were a favorite food of Emperor Caesar Augustus. A famous Sicilian legume dish, maccu, prepared with fava beans, was invented by Sicilian cooks in ancient times, enjoyed by people throughout the ancient Roman Empire, and still enjoyed today, simply prepared with fennel seeds and fava beans, olive oil, salt and pepper.

The first known school for professional cooks was created in Sicily and the documentation of its existence is given to us by Archestratus from Gela, a Greek poet from the 4th century BCE and who is considered the father of culinary critics.

Odysseus reports his admiration for the abundance of the Sicilian fields, beautifully described in the Odyssey (9th century BC). Plato discusses the Sicilian diet in his book, The Republic, as a diet rich in flavor which uses generous amounts of condiments and herbs. The first cookbook was written by Mithaceus of Syracuse in the 5th century B.C.

The Romans taught the Sicilians how to make sausages, how to prepare fish and how to collect and preserve the snow from Mount Etna, a large volcano on the east coast of Sicily. The Sicilians added honey and fruit juice to the fresh snow to create the first ice cream or "gelato". From the Romans they also learned how to dry fish by placing the fish in large containers under the sun to create anchovy paste that the Romans named Allex (thirst in Latin). Allex became the food of the peasants and slaves and it is still utilized today in the modern Sicilian cuisine.

The Sicilians also learned the art of preserving food in salt from the Romans. The "salsamantieri" were people whose job was to preserve food under salt that was exported all over the Roman Empire.

The Romans also taught the Sicilians how to make bread and the Sicilians perfected the art by adding seeds such as cumin, sesame and poppy. The Sicilian bakers made three types of bread, dark bread made from unrefined flour, a lighter colored bread named "panis secundaris" (the second bread), and "panis candidus" (white bread) made from refined flour that was favored by the wealthy. Bread making became an art and many different breads were created, in one recipe they added wine and honey to a bread that would eventually evolve into the famous Neapolitan Babà.

The following is a recipe from the book "De Re Coquinaria" by Marco Gavio Apicio, a Roman foodie, lover of condiments and luxury, that lived in the first century AD, during the Roman empire. This dish was commonly served in the Sicilian cuisine during the Roman time.

"ova fongia ex lacte" (four eggs, 27 ml of milk, 1 ounce of olive oil).

In 827 the Islamic conquest of Sicily began. The Arabs landed in the small town of Mazara Del Vallo situated less than 200 kilometers from north

Africa. In Sicily the Arabs did not create a unified Arabic reign but established several small lordships called kadi'.

The Christian communities in the central and western parts of the island resisted the Islamic acculturation. They were allowed to practice their religion as long as they paid a government tax. Palermo (Balarm in Arabic) was a very rich and opulent city under the Arabic domination. There were more than 300 mosques and a population of 250.000 habitants. (At that time the populations in Rome and Milan were each approximately 25,000.)

The Arabs left the greatest and most lasting impact on Sicilian food culture with the introduction of sugar cane, rice, citrus and spices. During the Arab domination, Sicily was considered the garden of the Mediterranean. As a result of the Arabic influence, by the year 1000 the Sicilian cuisine was more advanced and sophisticated than any other European cuisine.

The Sicilian cassata, cannoli, granite (Italian ice), sorbet and gelato were created during the time that the Arabs invaded the island. The Arabs also invented the first alcoholic beverages, however, since alcohol was forbidden by the Quran, it was used only for medicinal purposes.

During the Islamic conquest of Sicily, the Sicilians had mastered the art of pasta making and they exported pasta to several Muslims and Christian territories outside of Sicily.

The pasta dishes required the creation of sauces. It is believed that during the Arabic domination one chef was asked to feed the whole army. He created a pasta sauce made of sardines, wild fennel and pine nuts, "Mari e Monti" (sea and mountain, because of fish and fennel and pine nuts) which is still very much enjoyed in the modern Sicilian cuisine and utilizes carbohydrates, proteins and vegetables all in one dish. Some "malelingue" (gossiper) believe that the wild fennel was added to the sardines to mask the stench of old fish.

The immigration of Jews and others from the Middle East occurred at the same time that the Arabs colonized Sicily. The Jews in Sicily spoke an Arabic based language. Sicily at the time had 52 "giudecche", (Jewish neighborhoods) and 60 Synagogues.

The Ashkenazi Jews had a simpler cuisine and introduced broths, stuffed fish, potatoes and fruit compote into the Sicilian cuisine. The Sephardic Jews had a more elaborated cuisine like sweet and sour fish, meat and prune stew, carrot salad and cumin. The Sephardic Jews also introduced eggplant to the island and the Sicilians became experts in grilling, stuffing, frying and incorporating the purple fruit in pasta dishes such as "pasta alla Norma" which is one of our family favorites! (fresh tomato sauce, fried eggplant and salted ricotta cheese). This is the dish that above all others, tastes purely and sincerely like Sicily.

The Jews taught the art of Kashrut or Kosher which means eating appropriately. They introduced the concept of sautéing garlic in olive oil which added flavor in many dishes. They taught Sicilians how not to waste any food and how to utilize even the most insignificant parts of the animal they slaughtered (feet, tongue, liver, stomach, spleen,) an idea that has had recent resurgence in America today. Today, the street vendors in Palermo still sell "pani ca' meusa" (spleen and lung sandwich flavored with sesame.), as the Jews taught them many years ago. The Sicilian cuisine has a strong Arab-Sephardic Jewish influence.

The Normans were an ethnic group that arose in Normandy, the northern region of France, from contact between Viking settlers and indigenous Franks, the Gallo-Romans. In 1061 the Normans conquered Sicily. They landed in Messina, a town on the northeast coast of the Island, during a period of turmoil in the Arabic domination era of the island. At this time, several other populations from northern Europe also migrated to the island. The Normans reintroduced Christianity to Sicily and they constructed churches and monasteries. They converted most of the synagogues into churches.

The Normans greatly appreciated the Sicilian gastronomy. They brought to Sicily the art of drying fish (baccalà o Piscistoccu in Sicilian). Sicilians were very familiar with the art of cooking fish that was very abundant in the Mediterranean Sea, but they appreciated the dried fish for the ease of use and storage, and the high nutritious value. Today, during the winter months, when it is hard to go out at sea to fish, the Sicilians fish markets offer baccalà (dried cod fish) ready for sale as was taught to them by the Normans. The Normans also perfected the art of grilling game meat, which remains a Sicilian culinary art today.

The Normans also introduced eating utensils to Sicilian kitchens. In medieval times, very few owned knives. Guests would bring a spoon and a cup. The fork, introduced by the Normans, appears for the first time in the early XI century. The Spanish domination (1513-1714) introduced many new ingredients into the Sicilian cuisine, ingredients that had recently been imported from the Americas: tomatoes, peppers, potatoes, squash, prickly pear, turkey, cocoa, etc.

Sicilians were the first to farm tomatoes for consumption. The larger distribution of tomatoes to the rest of Europe would occur several centuries later, and remain a major export crop for Sicily today.

During the Spanish domination the eggplant parmigiana was created, now famous all over the world.

Pork was widely used and the "Pan di Spagna", angel cake, was created to improve the taste of the Sicilian Cassata cake. Sicilian "impanate" (empanadas), cooked mostly in the eastern part of Sicily were also introduced by the Spaniards.

The French occupied Sicily in the 1800s. From the French the Sicilians learned how to use onions instead of garlic in the preparation of refined sauces and the use of shortbread for dessert preparation.

In the 18th century the Sicilian aristocrats employed French cooks called " Monsù "(monsieur). The Monsù were often called by their first name and the last name of the noble families they worked for. Some of them became very famous and they occupied an entire apartment in the noble palace. The French and Sicilian cultures merged in the noblemen's Sicilian kitchens. The Sicilian peasant women that helped the noble families and the monsù, worked together to create a fusion cuisine that closed the gap between the two culinary cultures. This was a rare and unusual collaboration for that era. Together they created superb dishes that utilized the best of what the Sicilian land produced (farm to table). Many of their creations are still used today in the modern Sicilian cuisine, such as potatoes gateaux, rice timbales filled with meat, chicken stuffed with rice and giblets. These rich dishes are usually served, and deeply enjoyed, during a Sunday family dinner.

The peasant women that worked in the noble kitchens could not afford to buy meat for their family so they recreated the dishes they learned from the monsù by stuffing peppers and eggplants with rice instead of stuffing meats or they used sardines, which were abundant in the Mediterranean Sea, instead of chicken or game meat.

"Sarde a beccafico" (sardines stuffed with toasted bread crumbs, raisins, pine nuts, today recognized as one of the traditional Italian dishes), was the peasant womens' culinary version of stuffed game meat.

All of the many populations that conquered Sicily enriched the already rich Sicilian diet but did not alter its basic food preparation which continues to be practiced to this day. Nature and culture worked in synchrony to create one of the most diverse but coherent cuisines.

Sicily teaches us her history through the richness and variety of her food, a history that continues to represent itself in every Sicilian table and all over the world.

Our culinary traditions extend beyond the boundaries of Sicily but they have been protected inside this extraordinary island.

I am deeply grateful to all the women and men that have respected, loved, protected and cherished our gastronomic Sicilian tradition. It is through their love of our food that I can today share with my family and all of you the joy of preparing delicious food rich with excellent nutrition.

Fad Diets

OVER THE PAST 30 YEARS the western world has had to deal with the epidemic of obesity and fad diets have found a fertile environment to proliferate in. Vegan, api-vegan, raw vegan, macrobiotic, paleo, ketogenic, intermittent fasting, Mediterranean, pescatarian, pollo-pescetarian, omnivore, freegan, vegetarian, ova-vegetariano, lacto-ovo-vegetarian, fruitarian, juicearian, sproutarian, and carnivore are some of the fads. There are even breatharians who believe one can sustain themselves solely by the energy of the air and the universe!

Many of these diets are not based on science or traditions.

Short term diets almost never work and are not effective for lifelong well-being.

Short term crash diets are nutritionally depleted and can even cause heart disease.

(European Society of Cardiology (ESC). "Crash diets can cause transient deterioration in heart function." [2]

Fads and trends have resulted in malnutrition for many people. In the 1980s the American psyche was transfixed by what can only be described as fat phobia. The American Heart Association and the food industry joined in on the low-fat bandwagon and we ended up consuming increased amounts of refined carbohydrates. The truth of the matter is that healthy fats are necessary in our diets and eating sugars in excess proved very detrimental to our well-being. What followed was a disastrous epidemic of obesity, diabetes, and heart disease.

The gluten-free craze is another recent fad. Avoiding gluten is necessary for the very small group of people who have Celiac disease (1% of population) or have true gluten intolerance. For the rest of us, there is no evidence that eating a gluten-free diet promotes health. In fact, many packaged gluten-free products are inferior quality foods full of added sugar, added fat and added salt. A recent Harvard study found that people on a gluten-free diet eat less health-promoting whole grain foods.

Restrictive fad diets simply do not work. 95% of patients who go on a "crash" fad diet, gain all of the weight back in 1-5 years. The restrictive nature of crash diets leads to a diet-binge cycle, "yo-yo dieting", that has been shown to be deleterious for long term optimal health. Our bodies respond to crash diets by going into "starvation mode" and slowing down metabolism. In addition, fad crash diets are frequently lacking in essential nutrients. Starvation diets can be a trigger to developing eating disorders. There are thousands of weight loss supplements, fad diet books, and so-called celebrity "experts", all trying to capitalize on our desperation to lose weight. For example, the popular Atkins diet convinced millions that carbohydrates are a poison you must avoid at all costs while in fact whole grains are an essential part of a healthy diet. Recently the Paleo diet has suggested that we must follow the eating habits of our paleolithic ancestors, even though we do not really know what our paleolithic ancestors actually ate. The ketogenic (keto) diet, a high-fat, adequate protein, low-carbohydrate diet, is a new fad. In the 1920s this diet was used to treat epileptic children. The increased fat intake reduced the number of seizures they experienced. One of the problems with this diet is that it cannot be sustained for long periods, because our bodies need carbohydrates to stimulate insulin release for muscle growth. Therefore, one of the dangers of this diet is muscle loss, which is very hard to gain back. In addition, the reduction of quality carbohydrates results in an inadequate fiber intake creating constipation as a major side effect. This diet may increase heart disease, kidney disease and can be nutrient deficient because of the lack of phyto-nutrients, vitamins and minerals that are obtained only from a well-balanced diet.

Traci Mann, a psychology professor at University of Minnesota has studied why diets fail for over 20 years and published these findings in her book, "Secrets from the Eating Lab". Mann has observed that the biological changes that occur in our bodies because of dieting makes it almost impossible to keep the weight off. She does not believe that will power is the problem in achieving weight loss, but the changes in biology make diets fail. Mann believes that there are three important effects of diets that make weight loss impossible: the first is, that when we diet food looks more appetizing and it becomes harder to resist eating. The second is that diets create hormonal changes that instead of making us feel satisfied (satiety) they make us feel more hungry. Thirdly, when we are dieting metabolism slows down. The combination of these three factors work against us and make crash fad diets virtually impossible to work.

Our philosophy on nutrition is not have to reinvent the wheel as many of these fad crash diets are attempting to do. We have great examples of what actually works from our ancestors who are speaking to us. We do not have to try to imagine what our Stone Age ancestors were eating 2.5 million years ago. We do not have to eliminate entire classes of macronutrients which have been consumed healthfully by humans for thousands of years. What we should be doing is looking to the more recent past, more in line with our current genetic biology, and follow what has been shown to promote health. The Sicilian Secret way of eating is a style of eating that anyone can successfully maintain for their entire life.

Our goal in writing this book is to give readers a good sense of what a truly healthful diet is. As is outlined by Dr. Weston Price and Dan Buettner, if we only take the time to listen to what our ancestors are telling us, we can all live long and amazingly healthful lives.

Weston A. Price, DDS, author of Nutrition and Physical Degeneration and Dan Buettner, author of The Blue Zone Solution, are two researchers that have helped us to clarify how our ancestors have directed us onto a path of well-being by passing down knowledge of nutrition and lifestyle.

Weston A. Price, DDS, was a Cleveland dentist and is considered the father of modern nutrition research. Utilizing dental health as a marker of nutritional health, Dr. Price travelled the world in the 1930s studying the isolated human groups in Switzerland, Gaelic communities in the Outer Hebrides, Eskimos and Indians of North America, Melanesian and Polynesian South Sea Islanders, African tribes, Australian Aborigines, New Zealand Maori and Indians of South America.

Respectfully, he referred to these people as "primitive" because they were pure and untouched by modern civilization. What he found was that these people were free of chronic diseases, dental decay and mental illnesses.

Dan Buettner has identified the locations in the world (Blue Zones) where people frequently live to be 100 and older without experiencing chronic diseases such as heart disease, cancer, obesity or diabetes. These areas include Ikaria in Greece, Okinawa in Japan, Sardinia in Italy, Loma Linda in California, and Nicoya Peninsula in Costa Rica.

What these cultures all have in common is the fact that they strictly followed the nutritional advice handed down to them by their ancestors. Their diets were varied and included vegetables, fruits, meats, fish, poultry, legumes, nuts, seeds, raw foods, and whole grains. Their diets were free of processed foods or added sugar, salt and fats.

What is Special About *the* Sicilian Secret Mediterranean Diet?

IF WE TRULY WANT TO live longer and well we have to follow a diet that is simple and emphasizes the consumption of a variety of high quality and mostly plant based foods. We have learned to vilify large groups of macronutrients such as carbs and fats without understanding that there are "good" carbs and "bad" carbs and "good" fats and "bad" fats. The Sicilian Diet emphasizes the nutrients that are good for our health and delicious at the same time. For instance, The Sicilian Diet uses only good fats, the ones that are found in olive oil (monounsaturated fat) and in fish and nuts (polyunsaturated fats).

It is estimated that humans can live an average of an additional 25 quality years by simply improving lifestyle factors such as the quality of food, exercise, stress reduction and social networks. Healthspan is the number of quality disease-free years we live and lifespan is the actual number of years we live.

It is evident that the centenarians in these small Sicilian villages have optimized their genetic potential to the point of living well beyond the average life expectancy, increasing both their healthspan and lifespan. So, what is their secret?

First and foremost, Sicilians have adhered to the Sicilian version of a Mediterranean diet. This means that they consume mostly a plant-based diet, consisting of small portions of food eaten at three meal sessions with very little snacking between meals.

Their intake of meat is limited.

The bulk of calories consumed comes from seasonal fruits and vegetables.

This diet is naturally low in glycemic index or glycemic load which prevents the fast absorption of sugars and limits insulin spikes. The Sicilian Secret Diet is naturally anti-inflammatory.

The seasonality of food is important not only for plants but also for meats and cheeses. Foods are significantly more nutritious when they are in season, and since we have evolved alongside our friendly plants, our bodies have a circadian rhythm that metabolizes foods consumed in season much better than when they are not in season.

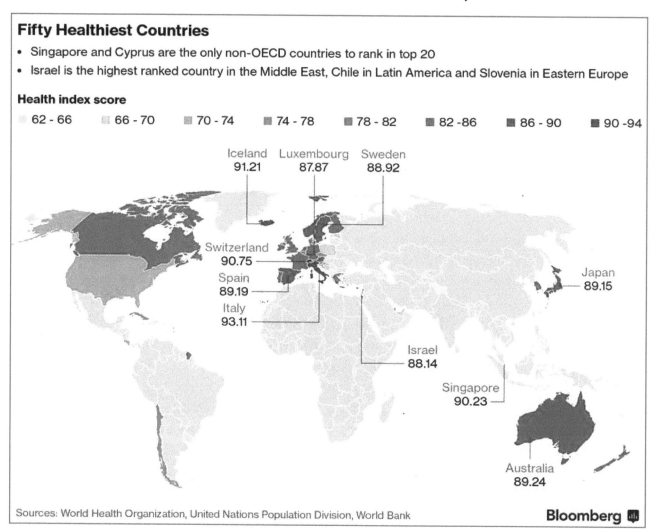

Fifty Healthiest Countries

- Singapore and Cyprus are the only non-OECD countries to rank in top 20
- Israel is the highest ranked country in the Middle East, Chile in Latin America and Slovenia in Eastern Europe

Health index score

| 62 - 66 | 66 - 70 | 70 - 74 | 74 - 78 | 78 - 82 | 82 - 86 | 86 - 90 | 90 - 94 |

Iceland 91.21
Luxembourg 87.87
Sweden 88.92
Switzerland 90.75
Spain 89.19
Italy 93.11
Japan 89.15
Israel 88.14
Singapore 90.23
Australia 89.24

Sources: World Health Organization, United Nations Population Division, World Bank

Bloomberg

How one combines foods is also important. In the Sicilian Secret Diet extra virgin olive oil is used in many dishes, and recent studies have shown that eating vegetables with oil promotes the absorption of fat soluble alpha and beta carotene, lutein, lycopene, two forms of vitamin E and vitamin K. These nutrients offer a wide range of health benefits, including cancer prevention and eyesight preservation. This is a great example of how the diverse food selection in the Sicilian Secret Diet promotes optimal wellness. [3]

Sicilian centenarians conduct a "low impact" life. What this means is that they exercise moderately but regularly throughout the day. In fact, many Sicilians, even in their advanced ages, are regularly walking to the market or standing in the kitchen preparing a meal. Rarely do they sit for any extended period of time.

We all would like to stay around as long as we can, feeling healthy, content and connected.

We have researched those studies that support the lifestyle changes that are necessary to achieve these goals.

U.S. News & World Report, 2018 best diets, places the Mediterranean diet in first place being associated with better overall health and longevity. We believe that the Sicilian Secret Diet is the best version of the Mediterranean Diet due to the depth and variety of the ingredients used in its cuisine.

The MEAL Trial (Mediterranean healthy Eating, Ageing, and Lifestyle) study - evaluated the total dietary intake of the beneficial compounds known as polyphenols in a group of Sicilian adults. Polyphenols are compounds that are found in foods common to the Sicilian Secret Diet such as vegetables, fruits, coffee, tea, olives, olive oil and wine. Researchers from the University of Catania, Sicily found that individuals with the highest intake of polyphenols had a 32% reduction in the risk of developing high blood pressure. When we ingest adequate quantities of Polyphenols the function of the inner lining of arteries, endotelium, improves. Polyphenols act in a similar manner to blood pressure drugs known as Angiotensin Converting Enzyme Inhibitors. I believe that you like me would much rather eat vegetables and fruit instead of taking medications to treat high blood pressure. [4]

Similar results were obtained in a recent research that demonstrated how a diet very similar to the Sicilian Secret Diet, The MIND Diet, helped to significantly slow the mental deterioration that occurs in survivors of brain attacks (strokes). MIND is a Mediterranean and DASH Diet (Dietary Approaches to Stop Hypertension) Intervention for Neurodegenerative Delay. [5]

Part I

THE FUNDAMENTALS

Chapter 1

WHY SAD IS BAD

The first step toward better health is knowledge

THE STANDARD AMERICAN DIET (SAD) *is* truly sad. The acronym tells the truth. The two leading causes of death in the U.S. (heart disease and cancer) are considered "lifestyle" diseases and diet is the biggest culprit. However, a good diet can prevent serious diseases and can reverse the ones that are already present.

Recent published research has shown that a nutritionally depleted Western Diet (SAD) can stimulate dormant (sleeping) cancer cells to come alive and kill. This is truly like waking the evil giant! ("Flipping the switch: Dietary fat, changes in fat metabolism may promote prostate cancer metastasis: Research reveals interplay between genes, environment in metastatic prostate disease.") [5]

People who are overweight cut their life expectancy by one month for every extra pound of weight. (According to a study from the University of Edinburgh who monitored over 6000,000 people). [6]

The obesity epidemic in the US accounts for almost 200,000 deaths annually. Childhood obesity has increased tenfold from 1975, (124 million last year compared with 11 million in 1975). [7]

Approximately 40 % of American adults and 18.5% of American children are obese. Michelle Obama started the national Let's Move campaign in 2010, but unfortunately the obesity rate in children has not gone down since. In the 1980s about 1 in 6 adults were obese. The rate climbed to 1 in 3 adults ten years ago and has not improved since.

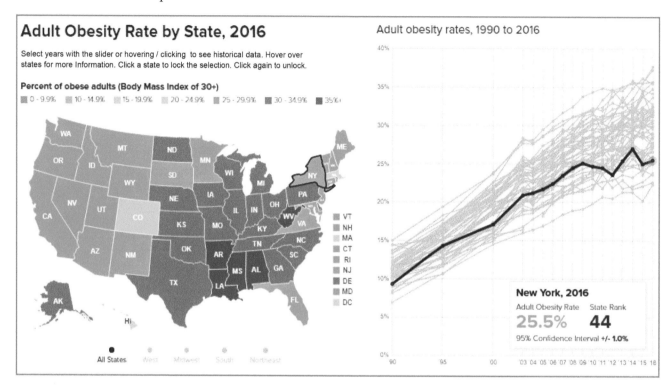

Adult Obesity Rate by State, 2016

Select years with the slider or hovering / clicking to see historical data. Hover over states for more Information. Click a state to lock the selection. Click again to unlock.

Percent of obese adults (Body Mass Index of 30+)

0 - 9.9%   10 - 14.9%   15 - 19.9%   20 - 24.9%   25 - 29.9%   30 - 34.9%   35%+

Adult obesity rates, 1990 to 2016

New York, 2016
Adult Obesity Rate   State Rank
25.5%   **44**
95% Confidence Interval +/- **1.0%**

Excessive processed meat consumption, typical of a Western SAD diet, increases breast cancer risk. Regular consumption of processed meat (the equivalent of half a hot dog) increased breast cancer risk in women by 20% [8]

On the other hand, research has shown that men who follow a Sicilian Secret Diet, rich in vegetables, whole grains, legumes, fish and olive oil lowered their risk for prostate cancer. These studies support that the same risk factors that cause heart disease can also cause cancers. Adhering to a healthful diet and lifestyle can both prevent and reverse disease. [9]

The typical SAD barely scores a 50 on a scale of 100 according to multiple data collected by the USDA Center for Nutrition Policy and Promotion, the

National Health and Nutrition Survey and a host of research findings published in leading medical journals.

That's an "F" on a school test.

For most Americans, more than 60 percent of the daily diet consists of refined carbohydrates, added fats, and added sugars—foods that are known to be harmful to health.

This low-quality diet has degraded the nation's health and has created an obesity epidemic. These nutritionally-depleted foods increase fat storage which is why approximately 65 percent of Americans are overweight and a third are obese.

It is well-established that diabetes, heart disease and cancer can result from being overweight or obese.

Of interest is a study that reports the findings from autopsies done on young American soldiers that were killed during the Korean and Vietnam wars. It showed that atherosclerosis was present in 80% of the soldiers. This shocking finding reveals that young men, mostly in their 20s, already have plaque in the coronary arteries. It is no wonder that there is an epidemic of heart disease in later life as these plaques continue to grow. [10]

Manifestations of coronary atherosclerosis in young trauma victims—an autopsy study.

Joseph A1, Ackerman D, Talley JD, Johnstone J, Kupersmith J.)

According to the Institute of Health Metrics and Evaluation, poor eating habits account for more deaths per year (approximately 700,000) than smoking (approximately 500,000 per year). The indirect effects of poor lifestyle choices are significant.

Yearly deaths from chronic diseases:

- **High blood pressure kills nearly 443,000 people.**

- **High body mass index kills 364,000.**

- **Physical inactivity kills 234,000.**

- **High blood sugar roughly 213,600.**

- **High cholesterol nearly 158,500.**

When we look at these numbers we know that we have to pay more attention to our children. They are more vulnerable to poor nutrition and have very little say in the choices of what they eat.

A recent study of 766 otherwise healthy adolescents found that those who consumed the least amount of vitamin K (found in spinach, cabbage, iceberg lettuce and olive oil) had a 3.3 time greater risk of developing heart disease. Vitamin K is very important for heart health and to promote healthy bones. American children eat very little of these health promoting foods that are abundant in the Sicilian Secret Diet. [11]

Low quality (junk) food leads to obesity in teenagers and has a negative effect on their brains, according to researcher Amy Reichelt, Ph.D. at RMIT University in Melbourne, Australia.

Since the brain is still developing during teenage years, eating a nutrient-poor junk food diet can negatively affect decision making by increasing reward-seeking behavior and influence poor eating habits throughout adulthood.

(Teratology Society. "Junk food, energy drinks may pose unique risks for teens, new data shows: Influences on teen brain development the focus of special Teratology Society journal issue." ScienceDaily, 18 December 2017.)

Healthy eating has been shown to be associated with increased happiness in children. Research has shown that healthy eating improves self-esteem and reduces peer problems. In addition, better self-esteem is associated to better adherence to healthy eating. So, teaching our children healthy eating habits can improve their overall well-being - a true gift. [12]

A study conducted in England confirms that children who eat take-out meals at least once weekly have higher body weight and higher bad (LDL) cholesterol compared to children who do not eat take-out meals. The same results are true for adults who regularly consume fast and take-out food. [13]

A single high fat meal causes transient high fat in the bloodstream (transient hypertriglyceridemia) which in turn causes stiffening and dysfunction of the very important inner lining (endothelium) of our blood vessels which can result in angina - chest pain - due to decreased blood flow to the heart muscle. [14]

That is why it is so important to eat healthy meals typical of the Sicilian Secret Diet that have been shown to improve the function of blood vessels and in doing so lower the risk of heart disease. [15]

The Sicilian Secret Diet has helped the elderly stay healthy and independent. In Sicily elders rarely go to nursing homes and tend to remain independent to a ripe old age. Weak and frail older adults have a hard time living independently and frequently become ill. There is evidence, however, that older people who adhere to the Sicilian Secret style Diet have a significantly lower risk of losing their independence because they are able to maintain muscle strength, activity, weight and energy levels.[16]

The epidemic of heart disease and other degenerative diseases is directly linked to our eating habits and lifestyle. In a certain sense we are victims of our wealth that provides us with readily available calories. Centenarians in Sicily consume small portions of food, mostly plant based. Meats are consumed in small quantities and everything including vegetables, fruits, meats, fish and cheeses are seasonally consumed.

An interesting phenomenon occurred in Norway during World War II. During the war most of the cattle was taken away and used to feed the German military. Therefore, the Norwegian population consumed almost no animal fat during those years. There was a significant decrease in the incidence of heart disease among the Norwegian population. When the war ended, and the beef and other animal products returned, the incidence of heart disease went right back to pre-war levels.[17]

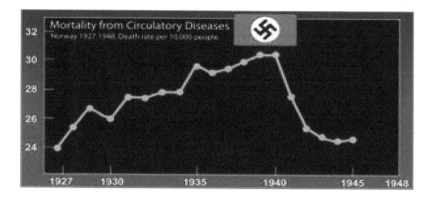

When I was a medical resident I was a researcher at the NIH Framingham Heart Study. I was involved in the landmark study that revealed how lifestyle factors are directly responsible for the development of heart disease. It has been shown that a diet low in animal protein results in lower inflammation, lower cancer risk, lower diabetes risk and lower overall mortality.[18]

Low animal protein intake is associated with a major reduction in inflammation, cancer, and overall mortality.[19]

Since 1950, Americans have been adding almost 70% more fats and almost 40% more sugar to their diets; they have been eating over 70 pounds of red meat per person per year, 65 pounds of chicken and fish yearly, and they have been consuming almost 1000 more total calories daily. Most Americans eat about 25 pounds of cheese per year which is found ubiquitously in many foods - pizza, Mexican food, sandwiches and salads. [20]

The low-carb fad began in 2000, however Americans continue to consume over 100 pounds of flour per year in the form of processed baked goods like donuts, bagels, muffins and pizza. The switch to healthy whole grains has not happened to any significant degree yet. Americans ingest almost 80 pounds of

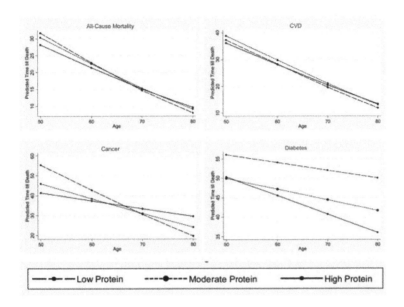

sugar per year mostly in the form of high fructose corn syrup added to sodas and juices.

Despite the push for low fat diets by government agencies and medical societies, the total added fats has risen from 30 pounds per person per year in 1970 to over 50 pounds today!

Vegetable consumption rose in the 1980s but has remained flat since and fresh fruit consumption has remained flat since 1970.

Americans are consuming significantly less whole milk, however the butterfat consumption has remained the same in the form of cheese used in different packaged and processed foods.

These trends explain why there are simultaneous epidemics of heart disease, obesity and diabetes. Heart disease is the number one cause of death for men and women, and the bigger tragedy is that it is preventable. We are victims of lobbyists and large corporations who have profits and not the health of the nation in mind.

The truth of the matter is that we do need regulations to protect consumers from poor corporate ethics. When food companies became mega international corporations, publicly owned, the focus moved away from producing healthy high quality food to producing profits on a 90 day cycle. Family run businesses can deal with a small profit margin, however large publicly owned companies need to show growth.

When former New York City Mayor Michael Bloomberg became frustrated with what was happening in his city, he took the first step of trying to reduce the size of sugary soda. Sodas are one of the principal ways food companies add sugar into American diets especially to low income Americans. Bloomberg's decision was criticized by many, especially food corporations, as an attack on personal freedom. The truth is that many Americans, and especially poor Americans live in "food deserts", far away from healthy markets but close to food marts full of soda and low quality, highly processed, packaged nutrient-poor foods. This creates a vicious cycle that can be interrupted only by providing education and government programs aimed to increase the quality of nutrition for Americans. In fact, the Green Market Program in NYC is a great example of how healthful foods can be brought successfully into low income neighborhoods. Our friend and colleague, Mr. Robert Lewis, helped create the system whereby food stamp users had a credit card instead of food stamps (which reduces the stigma associated with food stamps) and worked at changing the rules so that food stamp recipients could use their card to buy fresh fruits and vegetables from farmer's markets. This is the kind of forward thinking we need that can help people stay healthy. The Trump administration is trying to change the rules back so that food stamps can no longer be used in farmer's markets damaging both the consumer and the farmers.

The typical American diet is referred to as the SAD, because it is sadly bad for our health. We are a country of immigrants who came to America for the most part to escape poverty. As our country became richer the idea of bigger and more for less became the ethos for the average American. This may work for cars and electronics, but it is a disaster when it comes to food. The SAD is actually the opposite of a healthy diet. Foods loaded with saturated fats, salt, sugar and cheese are heavily consumed, while fiber and nutrient rich whole grains, vegetables, fruits, nuts, seeds and legumes, which promote health, are consumed in very small quantities. Research has shown that portion sizes make a big difference on the total calories consumed. Some single servings of food from chain coffee shops and fast food restaurants have as many calories as one should eat the entire day!

The ubiquitous presence of food makes it impossible to get away from the idea that we must eat something throughout the day. Instead of having our meals at home with our families, we now eat in the car, at our desk at work, in school, in libraries, in movie theaters, and even in churches. Some fast food chains have tried to introduce the concept of "the fourth meal" in an attempt to convince consumers that it is a good idea to eat four rather than three full meals daily. Many schools have sold their souls to soda companies and have walls of vending machines selling junk to our children. Remember, there is no such thing as junk food - it is either junk or food.

Humans have what I refer to as "nutritional intelligence" - the trillions of cells in our bodies need energy, and this is why we eat. When we eat nutrition dense foods we get satisfied (satiety) much sooner than when we eat nutrition poor (junk) foods. So, when we eat healthfully we can eat smaller amounts and feel satisfied. On the other hand, when we eat junk food we often do not feel satisfied because our cells are not receiving the nutrition they need and we continue to eat in a fruitless pursuit of nutrition, and the result is obesity, heart disease, diabetes and cancer. Many obese individuals are actually malnourished despite their extra pounds.

Our goal in this book is to provide guidance toward a better way of eating. What many people need to do is to re-train themselves to eat correctly.

The Sicilian Secret Diet can be practiced everywhere because plants, fruits, whole grains, good fats and healthy proteins are ubiquitously present. The recipes we present are delicious and easy to prepare.

The good news is that even small changes can make a significant difference in our health.

Chapter 2

IT'S NOT ENTIRELY YOUR FAULT

External factors that affect your nutritional health

Dominant Global Narrative

"It is not just Big Tobacco anymore. Public health must also contend with Big Food, Big Soda, and Big Alcohol."
-WHO Director General Margaret Chan

"Large companies that produce "junk food" are 21st C. pedophiles that violate the human rights of children."
-Chilean Senator, author of "stop sign" law

"With the scandal and outrage of the advertising and marketing of ultra-processed products to children, what's needed is resolute and even MILITANT action."
-Brazilian academic frequently cited by WHO and PAHO

The UN should negotiate a binding global convention "to curb the unchecked actions of powerful economic actors that have lately been flooding global markets with junk food."
-UN Special Rapporteur on the Right to Food

American Heart Association (AHA)

THE REASONS WE ARE FACING a growing epidemic of obesity, diabetes, and heart disease, may not be due to lack of character or willpower. We are influenced by outside factors beyond our control.

The AHA has recommended substituting animal fat with vegetable fat without the backing of good science. There are numerous studies that have put this recommendation into question. Butter from organic grass fed, non GMO, antibiotic-free cattle has been a healthy staple for our ancestors for thousands of years. For example, lard from grass fed pigs is full of healthy fat soluble vitamins. This idea that animal saturated fat is bad for us has resulted in the use of margarine (a butter substitute made from vegetable oils) in place of butter in schools, hospitals, and most US institutions.

The AHA has influenced other similar organizations around the world like the British Heart Foundation and the Australian Heart Foundation. The recommendation to eliminate animal saturated fats has resulted in increased consumption of refined carbohydrates and added sugars which in turn has raised triglycerides and has contributed to obesity, diabetes, and the metabolic syndrome. Additionally, the AHA has added its stamp of approval on products such as Honey Nut Cheerios (23 grams of refined carbohydrates, 10 grams of which is refined sugar), Quaker Instant Oatmeal with Maple & Brown Sugar (31 grams of carbohydrates, 12 grams of which is refined sugar) and V8 V Fusion (25 grams of sugar in one - as much as a soda). Millions of people buy products endorsed by the AHA under the false impression that these products promote health. This creates a problem on two levels. The first, is that we are told to eliminate all animal fats which includes good animal fats and the second is that we are substituting animal fat with low quality carbohydrates.

The root cause of diet related diseases is not high quality animal fat or high quality whole grains or high quality proteins but rather nutritionally depleted foods such as sugar, trans fats, and low quality cheese additives. These low quality foods are highly promoted by the food industry with direct advertising to children and adults. To make matters worse food companies pay to hide behind AHA endorsements which can be misleading to the general public. [21]

In 2014, Canada's Heart & Stroke Foundation announced that there is a need to wind back the "Health Check" program because its recommendations are promoting unhealthy choices. The Health Check program had previously placed its check of approval on things like margarine spreads, canola oil, mayonnaise (with flavors, artificial colors, and preservatives), and refined breads (with artificial flavors, msg, and artificial emulsifiers). However, the foundation, despite the recent dietary "awakening", continues to recommend that people consume margarine, vegetable and seed oils.

Sweden has become the first nation to develop national dietary guidelines that reject the idea that fats need to be substituted with carbohydrates. The Swedes believe that fats can be part of a nutritionally balanced healthy diet and that refined carbohydrates need to be reduced. The Swedish Council on Health Technology has stated that, "a high fat diet improves blood sugar levels, reduces triglycerides, and improves 'good' cholesterol, and has nothing but beneficial effects, including assisting in weight loss".

A recent study, the PURE Trial, revealed that whole fat dairy consumption resulted in reduced, not increased, heart disease. This study underscores the fact that when we consume quality foods there are many components of those foods that contribute to health. [22]

What we all need is more attention on lifestyle modification.

We know that poor lifestyle choices can lead to degenerative diseases like heart disease and cancer, and can be reversed with lifestyle changes such as diet and exercise. Pioneers like Dr. Dean Ornish and Dr. Caldwell Esselstyn have proven scientifically how lifestyle changes can be more powerful than drugs to reverse heart disease allowing patients to live a better quality of life. Americans need to create a better lifestyle culture that emphasizes exercise, rest, quality foods and time for love.

The French Lyon Heart Diet Study was one of the first studies that proved what constitutes a healthy diet. In this trial 605 heart attack survivors were assigned to eat either a Mediterranean-style diet (which includes quality animal fat, quality carbohydrates and quality protein) or a low-fat diet recommended by the AHA at the time. Four years later, the Mediterranean diet group showed to be 50-70% less likely to have repeat heart events and reported zero sudden deaths as compared to the low-fat AHA endorsed diet group! This was a more powerful effect than the ones obtained with the drugs we have available.

Recently, the AHA has recommended for Americans to reduce their sugar intake to 100-150 calories, but this may be a difficult suggestion for most people to adhere by, since sugar has so insidiously infiltrated our food supply. Our eating habits need to be a national priority and the AHA has an obligation to be at the forefront of this movement. [23]

It is apparent that in the past 30 years the efforts to reduce heart disease by substituting fat with refined carbohydrates has not worked. Cardiovascular disease, listed as the underlying cause of death, accounts for nearly 801,000.

I believe that it is important for all of us to have some understanding of how the institutions that have been created to protect us actually function.

The Food and Drug Administration (FDA) is an agency of the United States Department of Health and Human Services responsible for the safety and regulation of foods, dietary supplements, drugs, vaccines, biological medical products, blood products, medical devices, radiation-emitting devices, veterinary products and cosmetics. The FDA also enforces section 361 of the Public Health Services Act and the associated regulations, including sanitation requirements on interstate travel as well as specific rules for control of diseases on products ranging from animals sold as pets to donations of human blood and tissue.

The FDA was created in 1927 in order to carry out the Food and Drug Act put into effect by Theodore Roosevelt in 1906. In the 1900s unregulated medicines killed and injured many people. In addition, chemicals were added to spoiled food in order to mask their stench, so that it became necessary to regulate medicinals and food additives. The FDA was developed to help protect Americans from unscrupulous companies, unfortunately, recently the FDA has fallen short of its mission to help the well-being of Americans.

The FDA has been criticized by food safety experts for a variety of issues. Meat manufacturers use carbon monoxide gas mixtures during the packaging process to prevent discoloration of the meat - this technique may hide spoilage from consumers and prevents the meat from naturally turning brown. The FDA has banned the addition of food coloring, or color additives, explicitly for the reason that this may mislead the consumer to think that meat is fresher than it actually is.

("Some raising red flag over use of gas to keep meat in the pink". Pittsburgh Post-Gazette. February 19, 2006.)

Undoubtedly the FDA has protected Americans from many drugs, chemicals and medical devices. However, more recently the FDA is falling victim to the powers of big industry that put profits before safety. The FDA does not seem to properly investigate the conflicts of interest that researchers and doctors may have with clinical trials of drugs and medical devices. The New York Times article by Gardiner Harris (January 11, 2009) states; "In 42 percent of clinical trials, the agency did not receive forms disclosing doctors' financial conflicts and did nothing about the problem". He also added; "In 31 percent of the trials in which the agency did receive the required forms, agency reviewers did not document that they looked at the information".

The FDA has been accused of allowing the use of bovine growth hormone (rBGH) in dairy cows. Cows treated with rBGH secrete high levels of insulin-like growth factor 1 (IGF-1) in their milk and IGF-1 has been implicated in the growth of some cancers. The FDA approved rBGH in 1993, agreeing with industry that it is safe while all European Union countries maintain a ban on rBGH use due to the potential serious risks. A 1999 report by the European Commission Scientific Committee on Veterinary Measures relating to Public Health stated that scientific questions persist regarding the health risks of milk from rBGH treated cows, particularly for infants. [24]

The FDA allows for regular use of antibiotics in healthy domestic animals in order to facilitate the overcrowding of animals in "factory farms" and feedlots. These antibiotics are harmful to the animal and to the people who ingest the animal products and have contributed significantly to the epidemic of antibiotic-resistant strains of bacteria which further endangers the public. [25]

In August of 2013 the Pew Charitable Trust released a report that shows how the FDA allows the use of over 10,000 chemicals to be added to human food (pursuant to the Food Additives Amendment of 1958 and administered by the FDA.) According to this study the vast majority of these chemical have never been tested for harmful effects on humans. In fact, only 18% have good studies to support safety. The FDA has approved thousands of chemical additives before it defined safety or issued guidance establishing how a safety determination should be implemented. In one case in which the FDA approved hundreds of chemicals, the agency used "unwritten assumptions" and made safety decisions on "wish lists" submitted by industry, according to industry lawyers. [26]

Many additives fall into the category of GRAS (generally regarded as safe), however, as unbelievable as it may sound, the FDA allows for industry to state whether their own product is safe for human consumption without any toxicology studies to prove it. Once the FDA or an additive manufacturer determines a chemical "safe" to add to food, industry has little incentive to conduct further studies. In addition, the FDA does not systematically review its previous decisions. In 1997 the FDA launched the voluntary GRAS notification program - instead of the FDA independently assessing the safety of chemicals added to our food supply they rely on the "voluntary" opinion of the manufacturer!

The FDA has allowed for chemical additives such as coal tar derivatives to be used as food dyes (FD&C yellow 5 and 6 banned by most European countries). Certain additives can cause cancer and have been associated with hyperactive behavior in children, but the manufacturers find them to be "generally regarded as safe" (GRAS). (Looking Back to Look Forward: A Review of the FDA's Food Additives Assessment and Recommendations for Modernizing its Programs. [27, 28]

In a 2011 policy statement the American Academy of Pediatrics condemned a 1976 law that allows for chemical manufacturers to "self-regulate" their own products. The Toxic Substance Control Act actually limits federal officials from ordering testing or banning industrial chemicals. Dr. Jerome Paulson, a Washington D.C. pediatrician and the lead author of the academy's statement stated, "we share the frustration of a lot of people that these chemicals are being addressed with sort of a flavor-of-the-month approach". Under current law, the U.S. Environmental Protection Agency and the FDA acknowledge that they know little about thousands of chemicals produced (1 million pounds a year or more) to which we are all exposed including our children. There are many indirect and direct ways that children are exposed to these potentially toxic chemicals, such as sucking on toys, drinking from plastic bottles, or playing on chemically treated carpets and there are many studies demonstrating that children are absorbing a great number of these harmful substances. Manufacturers are not required to disclose their ingredients and our government agencies respond by stating that confidentiality rules prevent them from sharing information with the public they are supposed to protect.

Despite all of this data on BPA the FDA remains ambiguous.

The FDA, which is responsible for ensuring the safety of most of the U.S. food supply, is not required to review spices and preservatives that are added to foods that are generally regarded as safe (GRAS). Currently, companies may determine a substance is GRAS without the FDA's approval or knowledge. However, substances previously considered GRAS have been banned. In 2010 the Government Accountability Office (GAO) reported that the FDA is not ensuring the safety of many chemicals.

Engineered nanomaterials, which are manufactured particles microscopic in size, enter the food supply as GRAS substances without FDA oversight. Because GRAS notification is voluntary and companies are not required to identify nanomaterials in their GRAS substances, the FDA has no way of knowing the full extent to which engineered nanomaterials have entered the U.S. food supply.

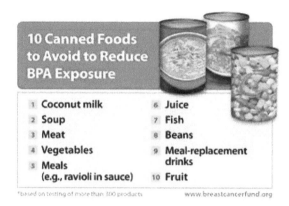

10 Canned Foods to Avoid to Reduce BPA Exposure

1 Coconut milk
2 Soup
3 Meat
4 Vegetables
5 Meals (e.g., ravioli in sauce)
6 Juice
7 Fish
8 Beans
9 Meal-replacement drinks
10 Fruit

*based on testing of more than 300 products   www.breastcancerfund.org

In contrast, all food ingredients that incorporate engineered nanomaterials must be submitted to regulators in Canada and in the European Union before they can be marketed.

Dr. Michael Hansen, a senior scientist at Consumers Union has stated that many additives in our food system are never tested for safety. Hansen also added that he does not put much faith on when a company designates their product as GRAS. Moreover, these potentially toxic chemicals when used in combination can become even more toxic. A study conducted in 2006 (Synergistic interactions between commonly used food additives in a developmental neurotoxicity test. Toxicology Science 2006 Mar; 90(1):178-87) concluded that the combination of several common additives appear to have a neurotoxic effect. In another study (Synergistic effects of food colors on the toxicity of 3-amino-1, 4-dimethyl-5H-pyrido [4,3-b] indole (Trp-P-1) in primary cultured rat hepatocytes. Journal of Nutritional Science and Vitaminology 2000 Vol. 46 No. 3 pp. 130-136) researchers found that the combination of four major food additives or six common food colors caused toxicity. Alone, each of the additives and food colors are considered "GRAS" by the manufacturer. Another study (Synergistic Toxicity of Food Additives in Rats Fed a Diet Low in Dietary Fiber. Journal of Food Science Vol 41, Issue 4, pp. 949-951, July 1976) looked at three common food additives - while any one was not significantly toxic, the combination resulted in weight loss and death of all of the test animals. [29, 30, 31]

Most processed foods contain many additives. Seemingly benign foods can hide potentially harmful chemicals - for instance, a Subway sandwich of turkey and cheese with fat-free honey mustard, peppers and pickles contains more than 40 different food additives, preservatives and dyes. A simple item like Dannon Light & Fit yogurt contains over 12 different chemical additives. Dr. Hansen, of Consumers Union, believes that many Americans routinely consume over 100 chemical food additives daily. The health effects and the synergistic negative health effects are difficult to measure, but undoubtedly they contribute to the epidemic of chronic degenerative disease that are making Americans sick every year.

Our bodies absorb significant amounts of chemicals through the skin and through the lungs when we use personal care products such as shampoos, soaps, lotions, and cleaning products. A recent study (Toxic Effects of the Easily Avoidable Phthalates and Parabens. Altern Med Review. 2010 Sep; 15(3):190-6) found that phthalates and parabens which are frequently utilized in personal care products, foods and household dust, can cause infertility, testicular dysgenesis, obesity, asthma, allergies, leiomyomas (a cancer) and breast cancer. These substances are estrogen-like and therefore of particular significance for breast cancer risk.[32]

Trans Fats

It is no longer a question that trans fats in any amount are deleterious for our health. Trans fats are artificial food additives made by adding hydrogen to vegetable oils which turns liquid oils into solid fat. Originally this was done to reduce cost - corn oil made solid was cheaper than butter or lard. Paradoxically hydrogenation destroys the healthy omega-3 fatty acid! Trans fats are commonly found in microwave popcorn, frozen pizza, coffee creamers, cookies, cakes and many other products. Dr. Walter Willet (Intake of trans fatty acids and risk of coronary artery disease among women. Lancet. 1993 Mar 6;341(8845): 581-5) showed that trans-fat increases the risk of heart disease. Dr. Walter Willet, the Frederick John Stare Professor of Epidemiology and Nutrition and chair of the Department of Nutrition at the Harvard School of Public Health has stated; " trans fats are the biggest food processing disaster in U.S. history, causing up to 100,000 premature deaths annually from heart disease". Because of significant push back from the food industry the FDA was easily manipulated to delay the ban of trans fats for decades, resulting in avoidable deaths from heart disease. In 2006 the FDA required listing of trans fats on nutritional labels and allowed for products that contain less than 0.5 grams of trans fats to be labeled as "no trans fats". No amount of trans fats in the diet is safe.

Of particular annoyance to me as a nutritional cardiologist is Benecol. Benecol is advertised as a health promoting cholesterol-lowering food because it contains plant sterols. It states no trans fats, but partially hydrogenated soybean oil (trans fat) is listed as an ingredient. What is the use of trying to lower cholesterol with plant sterols when trans fats will increase the risk of heart disease? [33]

In 1975 Dr. Benjamin Feingold, "Why Your Child is Hyperactive", raised the idea that food dyes cause Attention Deficit Hyperactivity Disorder (ADHD). In 2007 and 2010 researchers at the University of Southampton in the United Kingdom found that food dyes and sodium benzoate (a food preservative) increase ADHD symptoms in both hyperactive and non-hyperactive children. The FDA advisory committee has established that there is insufficient evidence to support a link between artificial dyes and ADHD. The FDA allows for eight dyes in the U.S. - Citrus Red 2, Red 3, Red 40, Blue 1 & 2, Green 3, and Yellow 5 and 6. These dyes have no nutritional values. [34]

FDA Commissioner Margaret Hamburg has testified before lawmakers that the agency feels "comfortable" with a 1992 policy that states food made with genetically modified organisms (GMO) are not materially different from non-GMO foods. Hamburg has stated; "We have not seen evidence of safety risks associated with GMO foods."

Unfortunately GMO products are already present in over 80% of our food supply.

Ronnie Cummins, the national director of the Organic Consumers Association stated; "it is an insult to anyone who buys food in this country to go on record stating that the FDA has 'not found evidence of safety risks' associated with GMO's". Cummins pointed out the statement signed by 300 scientists and doctors saying there is "no scientific consensus on GMO safety."

In an effort to circumvent GMO labeling legislation, food industry groups, such as the Grocery Manufacturers Association, have proposed a "voluntary" labeling system which would be linked to a ruling that would ban states from passing mandatory labeling regulations.

Louis Finkel, the Grocery Manufacturers Association executive vice president for government affairs stated; "there is no material difference between genetically engineered ingredients and their conventional counterparts".

The Center for Food Safety in 2011 submitted a petition calling upon the FDA to issue regulations requiring mandatory labeling. Sen. Barbara Boxer (D-Calif) sponsored legislation that would direct the FDA to enact regulations imposing mandatory labeling.

In order to help bring some balance to this issue U.S. Representative Ron Paul introduced a bill on November 10, 2005 titled the "Health Freedom Protection Act" (H.R. 4282), which proposes to stop "the FDA from censoring truthful claims about the curative, mitigative, or preventative effects of dietary supplements, and adopts the federal court's suggested use of disclaimers as an alternative to censorship." (http://www.lewrockwell.com/paul/paul288.html "Free Speech and Dietary Supplements") [35]

Herbert L. Ley, M.D. was appointed Commissioner of the Food and Drug Administration by President Lyndon B. Johnson on July 1, 1968. After his resignation, in a New York Times interview, he warned the public about the FDA's inability to protect the consumers. He stated that he was constantly pressured by industries to approve drugs and chemicals for the interest of profits and not safety. Dr. Ley's famous quote upon his resignation, "The thing that bugs me is that people think the FDA is protecting them - it isn't. What the FDA is doing and what the public think it's doing are as different as night and day".

Western Medicine

I wanted to be a doctor from as far back as I can remember - I think I was six years old and my father, who was an old time general practitioner, took me with him on house calls. Even at that young age I could see that my father's mere presence made his patients feel better.

Medicine is much more than an accumulation of knowledge - it is the understanding that the patient is greater than the illness he or she presents. Both the body and the human need attention and nurturance. Medical schools in the United States are now starting to add the teaching of lifestyle medicine to their medical students with the inclusion of nutrition, stress reduction, meditation and yoga.

There is a lot that is not understood in medicine. Since our bodies are composed of trillions of cells, and each of these cells perform thousands of chemical reactions per second, we will never really understand the many mysteries of the human body. Medicine is an inherently imperfect science.

Healing is both a science and an art. Central to the success of a good healer is the ability to listen to patients, understand their fears and respond to their true desires for wellness.

Many of the therapies used in modern day Western medicine were discovered and developed during war times. This way of providing medical care (referred to as allopathic medicine) is very effective for acute care medicine. US hospitals are capable of dealing with emergencies with prompt efficacy.

The problem with our system is that the majority of illnesses people face today are not acute care emergencies, but rather chronic degenerative diseases such as heart disease, cancer, diabetes, obesity, metabolic syndrome, arthritis and other conditions that require a different approach from acute care.

Life expectancy in the US is 78.9 years, which is ranked as 58th in the world. This is the lowest ranking since we started keeping track in 1970.

Every year over 700,000 Americans have a heart attack (http://circ.ahajournals. org/content/127/1/e6.long), and the cost of coronary artery disease alone in the United States is over $100 Billion each year. [36]

Cardiovascular diseases

Cardiovascular disease is the leading cause of death in the United States and is responsible for 17% of the total national healthcare expenditure. By 2030, 40.5% of the US population is projected to have some form of heart disease. The direct medical costs from heart disease is projected to triple from $273 billion in 2010 to $818 billion in 2030. The indirect cost due to lost productivity is estimated to increase from $172 billion in 2010 to $276 billion in 2030. The total costs in 2030 is estimated to be over $1 trillion!

The British Orbita Trial looked at a very commonly performed procedure, coronary angioplasty and stenting. 600,000 angioplasties are performed in the U.S. each year at a cost of over $12 billion, and the risks of the procedure include heart attack and possible death. Heart stents are most often used to treat angina - chest pain that occurs when physically active. The study was divided in two groups, in one group the patients received a stent and in the other group the patients received a "sham" procedure (they did not receive a stent).

There was no significant difference in the reduction of angina between those who received a stent and those who did not receive a stent. Many reasons have been postulated to explain this finding, including that atherosclerosis is a diffuse process and stent only takes care of the blockage in the large part of the artery, while most patients who have angina have diffuse disease in the small arteries downstream to the stent which is not improved by the stenting procedure.

Atherosclerosis, blockages of the heart arteries and arteries throughout the body is a "lifestyle" disease, meaning that the disease is a consequence of our poor choices - diets, exercise, stress, and other reversible risk factors.

There is excellent scientific data collected by pioneers in lifestyle medicine such as Dr. Dean Ornish and Dr. Caldwell Esselstyn, that have shown how a lifestyle change creates powerful improvements in our health. The Sicilian Secret Diet is a version of a lifestyle change that can be easily implemented that will add joy to your life and will improve your health. [37]

We can reverse heart disease!

Minimizing meat and dairy, avoiding refined sugar and processed foods, increasing vegetables, fruits, legumes, whole grains, will move patients away from a state of disease and toward a state of health, according to an article published in the Permanente Journal. More than 20 clinicians authored a report that reviewed lifestyle changes that could decrease premature disability and death. They caution that healthcare professionals should be informing their patients of the root causes of chronic diseases, and that many diseases are not inevitable but rather preventable and even reversible with healthy lifestyle interventions, including dietary changes, physical activity, and stress management. [38]

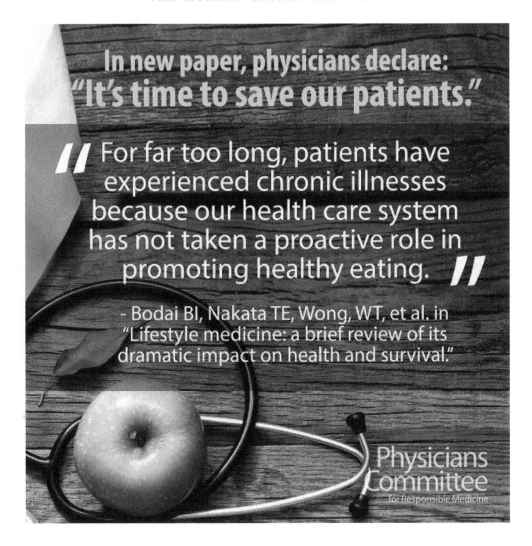

In new paper, physicians declare: "It's time to save our patients."

" For far too long, patients have experienced chronic illnesses because our health care system has not taken a proactive role in promoting healthy eating. "

- Bodai BI, Nakata TE, Wong, WT, et al. in "Lifestyle medicine: a brief review of its dramatic impact on health and survival."

Physicians Committee for Responsible Medicine

The US spends more on healthcare than any other nation on the planet. We have reached a tipping point in this country where we spend more on healthcare than we do on food! The reasons that we spend about an extra $2000 per person as compared to other industrialized countries is varied and complicated, unfortunately, we do not receive better care with this extra expense.

Market forces are at work aiming to sell a drug for every part of our hearts. Lipitor is a good example of these market dynamics. Lipitor (brand name) or atorvastatin (generic name) is in the statin class of cholesterol lowering drugs. Lipitor came onto the market in 1997 in a crowded field with 5 other drugs, three of which were blockbusters which already accounted for over $1 billion a year in sales. Lipitor would become the top selling drug of all time, with over $125 billion in sales in the ensuing 15 years!

Lipitor was initially developed by Warner-Lambert and then subsequently sold to Pfizer. The timing for the release of Lipitor could not have been better - For the first time in 1997 The Food and Drug Administration allowed direct-to-consumer advertising. At the same time medical associations kept lowering the recommended cholesterol targets. So Pfizer took full advantage and spent tens of millions on advertising. It advertised during the popular medical drama "ER", urging viewers to "Know Your Numbers" and then showing how easy it can be to get the cholesterol numbers below the guideline goals utilizing Lipitor. Pfizer underwrote over 400 studies together with some of the most prestigious medical schools and hospitals in the country, which included over 80,000 patients and cost over $1 billion. Pfizer spends over $3 billion every year on promotion and advertising.

We can only wonder what could happen if we spent that amount of money on lifestyle modification - teaching people how to eat properly, how to maintain optimal weight, how to reduce stress, and how to exercise. We do know, however, based on the work of Dr. Caldwell Esselstyn and others, that lifestyle modification is more effective in lowering cholesterol than statins. There are serious side effects of statins - muscle pain (myopathy), liver function abnormalities, dementia and diabetes, just to name a few. Former astronaut, Dr. Duane Graveline, has written a book, "Lipitor: Thief of Memory", about his loss of memory secondary to Lipitor Lifestyle change is not only side effect free it has side benefits. This is not to say that high risk patients should not take statins - if you have suffered a heart attack, had a heart stent or coronary bypass surgery you are at elevated risk and statins are an appropriate adjunct, especially if one cannot optimize life-style factors. For many patients, especially for primary prevention (those patients without known heart disease) an improvement in lifestyle is the most important factor to prevent disease.

David Rothman, who studies conflicts of interest in medicine at Columbia University, believes that societies that represent specialists welcome financial input from industry. These societies, like the Heart Rhythm Society, accepts nearly half of its $16 million operating budget from the makers of drugs, cathe-ters, defibrillators, pacemakers and many other companies. The problem is that these societies are a very important part of healthcare implementation - they write national guidelines, lobby Congress, and are essential sources of informa-tion for both healthcare practitioners and the public. So, behind the smokescreen of a national professional society, doctors wittingly or unwittingly are agents for industry. There is a lot of money at stake. A single implantable defibrilla-tor - a device that when used appropriately is life-saving by shocking a diseased heart back to a normal heartbeat - can cost over $30,000. The cardiologists who specialize in these devices will implant dozens per year based on the guidelines written by their specialty society, which is funded by the companies that make the device.

There is some movement for more transparency for professional societies and their ties to industry.

As evidence that industry is actually influencing the over utilization of these devices, an article in the Journal of the American Medical Association found that over 20% of patients who received implanted defibrillators did not meet the medical evidence-based criteria for their use. [39]

A Japanese pharmaceutical company that makes four high blood pressure drugs, Daiichi Sankyo, paid the American Society of Hypertension(ASH) about $2000 for each of its 1200 drug representatives to be trained and to print the ASH Accreditation symbol on their business card. So, each representative will hand the doctor his or her business card with the ASH stamp of approval.

This would insinuate that the particular drug is backed by ASH and eventually will lead to either over-utilization or to use more expensive brand name drugs in place of cheaper and equally effective generic drugs. According to Sen. Grassley's investigation, Daiichi gave the American Society of Hypertension more than $3.3 million.

In a perfect world there would be no financial motives for providers when it comes to the health of a person. Most doctors strive to do the right thing for their patients, unfortunately, they may have been unwittingly influenced by the medical industrial complex. Most healthcare providers are inadequately trained in nutrition and lifestyle medicine and are not allotted the time needed to counsel patients on ways of naturally preventing and reversing disease.

The lifestyle approach to medical care that uses natural, holistic, and integrative modalities, places the patient at the center of the care as an active participant in the decision making. The patient needs to guide the care and collaborate with his or her health care practitioners in order to achieve balance and wellness.

Sir William Osler: "If you listen carefully to the patient, they will tell you the diagnosis".

Food Industry

Large food companies must advertise excessively in order to grow. The goal is to get people to eat a large quantity of refined foods with cheap and unhealthful additives so they increase portion sizes and create new and "improved" products that consumers will buy more of. Of particular concern is the direct marketing to children that is allowed in America and is banned in many other countries.

In the 1990s the US government created the Food Labeling Act which required that food companies label foods with all ingredients. As a compromise the food companies were allowed to make health claims on their packaging. This eventually took on a life of its own with food companies competing with each other, making misleading and wildly exaggerated claims about the health benefits of their particular product. For example, when the medical community decided that fat was bad, food companies produced thousands of "low fat", "reduced fat" and "fat-free" products. In many of these products, the fat was substituted with sugar, artificial sweeteners and many different chemical additives. Consumers unfortunately buy products with these misleading claims under the false belief that these are "healthy" foods.

"Whole grain", "natural fruit flavor", and "antioxidants" are examples of marketing tricks designed to make the consumer purchase a product that has very little of that particular ingredient. A processed bread made mostly from refined flour with a sprinkle of whole grain, has essentially none of the benefits of whole grain, but "Whole Grain" will be found in large print on the package. Products that boost "natural fruit flavor" frequently have insignificant amounts of fruit and significant amounts of sugar and artificial flavors and coloring. Products that state "antioxidants" are banking on your knowledge that antioxidants are good for you but the amount of antioxidants added is so small that it will hardly have a beneficial health effect.

Another trick of food companies is to name things in ways that they may not be readily recognized. For instance, sugar is sometimes called sugar, but it is also called evaporated cane sugar and high fructose corn syrup. A particular food product may have all three of these ingredients, which are different names for the same thing - sugar! Processing food and adding sugar makes the food more profitable but also makes the food nutritionally depleted with negative health effects.

A frequent advertising ploy by food companies is to promote the latest food fad on the product. Food companies are well aware of all of the trends in eating that may potentially be a marketing opportunity. Statements like "low carb", "gluten-free", "low-fat", "zero calories" are designed to attract one to buy the product. These products are frequently complete junk from a nutritional standpoint.

As awareness of the obesity epidemic increases, food companies have become more creative in their tactics. They have invented fake grill marks on pre-packaged burgers and other natural "looks" to their products, all designed to make consumers think they are getting a more "natural" or more "artisanal" food.

Advertising to children should be banned in all its forms

Childhood obesity is increasing dramatically and some children are actually undergoing liver transplants for fatty livers due to excessive sugar intake. According to some estimates by the Federal Trade Commission and other entities, food makers spend between $1.6 and $10 billion on advertising to children. Food companies have reported their half-hearted reductions of food advertising to children to the FCC, however, they have not reported their ramped up efforts in advertising food to children on the Internet, social media outlets and children's video games. These newer forms of advertising are unregulated and more effective than traditional marketing. The average child downloads approximately 30 apps a year and 30% of 5 to 15 year olds own a smartphone. 28% of preschoolers can use a smartphone app while only 11% can tie their shoelaces! The popular Cooking Mamma app emphasizes sugary junk food. "Advergames" use smartphone games to promote junk and fast food - Burger King has partnered with the popular game, "Cut The Rope" and McDonald's has partnered with "Angry Birds".

The average child in the US watches 15 food commercials per day or (over 5500 per year) on television. The Joe Camel campaign aimed to get kids to smoke was clearly criminal, today, however, we allow cartoon characters to encourage our children to consume nutritionally depleted, obesity-promoting junk food. In the 1950s half of Americans smoked. We are now in a similar stage with food companies as we were with tobacco companies in the 1950s. Additives, like trans fats and sugars should be considered as toxic and as addictive as tobacco and marketing to children should be banned in all it's forms.

McDonald's French fries made in the US contain over 12 additives including trans fats, Sodium Acid Pyrophosphate to maintain color and Dimethylpolysiloxane as an anti-foaming agent. McDonald's French fries made in the UK contain only potatoes, vegetable oil and salt.

Kellogg's Smart Start Strong Heart Antioxidants has a name that promotes health, however it contains BHT (butylated hydroxytoluene), high fructose corn syrup, artificial vanilla flavor, and Yellow #5. The National Toxicology Program has identified BHT as a probable human carcinogen. High Fructose Corn Syrup has a very high glycemic index, leads to obesity and diabetes and is produced from genetically modified corn and frequently contains mercury. Yellow #5 is produced from coal tar and is also a potential cancer causing agent.

Other additives such as propylene glycol alginate (E405), polysorbate 60, soybean oil and many others are routinely added to seemingly healthy processed foods like salad dressings, snacks, and even some veggie burgers.

The article "Molecular basis for the herbicide resistance of Roundup Ready crops", Proceedings of the National Academy of Science of the United States of America vol 103(35); 2006 Aug 29, shows how Monsanto created a way to inhibit an enzyme which makes plants resistant to the herbicide Roundup. Roundup chemicals are used ubiquitously throughout the US - it is found in big cities like New York City to the smallest rural town. It is utilized on lawns and over 8000 tons are utilized on all sort of crops.

Monsanto manufactures both the Roundup and the seeds that are genetically modified to be resistant to the herbicide. This means that farmers can liberally utilize Roundup to kill weeds and the cash crop will not be affected. On the surface, this may sound like a great advance, however, it has resulted in many problems for our health and for the environment. Roundup has been linked to Parkinson's disease, infertility, cancer and heart disease. The principal ingredient in Roundup is glyphosate and is the most popular herbicide worldwide. Glyphosate has been found in foods we regularly ingest. Monsanto insists that glyphosate is harmless to humans, however, Anthony Samsel and Stephanie Seneff of

MIT published in the journal ENTROPY, that glyphosate enhances the damaging effects of other food borne chemical residues and environmental toxins.

("Anthony Samsel and Stephanie Seneff, "Glyphosate's Suppression of Cytochrome P450 Enzymes and Amino Acid Biosynthesis by the Gut Microbiome: Pathways to Modern Diseases" Entropy 2013, 15(4), 1416-1463; doi:10.3390/e15041416 (Download)–See more at: http://naturalsociety.com/dr-stepha-nie-seneff-mit-scientist-explains-synergistic-effect-aluminum-glypho-sate-poi-soning-cause-skyrocketing-autism/#sthash.wCqjyA9p.dpuf)

Dr. Seneff also believes that glyphosate could be associated with the skyrocketing rates of autism in the US. The way glyphosate works is by interrupting the shikimate pathway, a plant metabolic pathway that creates essential amino acids - when this pathway is disrupted the plant dies. Monsanto claims that humans and their genetically modified plants do not have a shikimate pathway, therefore, glyphosate is harmless to humans. As it turns out, humans do have a shikimate pathway which helps our body to eliminate poisons like Roundup and other herbicides and pesticides. Bacteria also have a shikimate pathway, so Roundup can cause havoc on our gut friendly bacteria. This results in a leaky gut, decreased immunity and the development of diseases associated with inflammation such as heart disease. In the presence of glyphosate, aluminum, which is very toxic to humans, is absorbed and accumulates instead of being expelled. [40]

Moms Across America are trying to fight giant agra companies such as Monsanto. Glyphosate is found in drinking water in America (ten times the amount allowed in European drinking water!), in blood and even in breast milk.

Moms Across America have drafted a petition to the Centers for Disease Control and Prevention and the Food and Drug Administration, demanding further testing and regulation of glyphosate:

"Considering the CDC's and FDA's mission to 'protect American health', we Moms and supporters ask the CDC and FDA to remain true to your commitment and to immediately conduct and require LONG-TERM AND LIFETIME

tests to determine if there is any risk or danger to our citizens and children by genetically modified foods and their required herbicides and pesticides such as Glyphosate (Roundup), Bt Toxin, 2,4-D, Dicamba, Glufosinate etc.

We believe the systemic reason (for increased disease and ill health in the U.S.) is that, unlike other countries, 80% of the food in the US contains ingredients from genetically modified crops that contain foreign proteins and has been doused in glyphosate herbicide which has been shown to damage the beneficial bacteria in our gut which is the stronghold of our immune system. Glyphosate also impairs the liver's ability to detox and breaks down the blood brain barrier to allow toxins into the brain."

The American College of Obstetrics and Gynecologists and the American Society for Reproductive Medicine have issued joint statements urging the EPA to limit chemicals such as glyphosate that can negatively impact a woman's ability to have children.

A New York Times poll reported that 93 percent of respondents support a GMO labeling law. Initiative 522 is a Washington State ballot measure created in order to permit GMO labels and proposition 37 in California is a similar movement. The Grocery Manufacturers of America, composed by powerful members such as Monsanto, Conagra, General Mills, Campbell's Soup Company, Kellogg Company, Land O'Lakes, Ocean Spray, Cargill, Dean Foods, Unilever, The Hershey Company, Bayer CropScience, Dupont, Coca-Cola, Pepsi and Nestle have poured tens of millions of dollars in both states to defeat these measures.

Wood, or cellulose, appears on the ingredient list as cellulose gum, powdered cellulose, microcrystalline cellulose, methyl cellulose, carboxymethyl cellulose, sodium carboxymethyl cellulose, hydroxypropylmethyl cellulose, ethyl cellulose, and cellulose acetate. J. Rettenmaier USA, a large manufacturer of cellulose for plastics, cleaning detergents, welding electrodes, cat litter, automotive brake pads, glue, asphalt and paints also makes "organic" cellulose for processed foods for both human and animal consumption. Cellulose is water-absorbing, so that the cellulose-water combination becomes an inexpensive filler for processed foods. Wood pulp is added to ice cream, salad dressings, barbecue sauces and many other foods. According to the FDA cellulose is safe for human consumption and has placed no limits on the amount of cellulose that can be added to food. By the FDA's own reporting methyl cellulose causes maternal mortality and retardation of fetal maturation in mice (Select Committee on GRAS Substances (SCOGS) Opinion: Carboxymethyl cellulose)

Acrylamide is a toxic ingredient frequently found in processed foods, especially chips, baked goods and French fries. It is a cancer-causing neurotoxic agent. The FDA limits acrylamide in drinking water to 0.5 parts per billion, or about 0.12 micrograms in a glass of water. French fries can contain up to 60 micrograms of acrylamide or over 500 times above the allowable FDA limit. In a 2005 report by the California-based Environmental Law Foundation (ELF), "How Potato Chips Stack Up: Levels of Cancer-Causing Acrylamide in Popular Brands of Potato Chips", they found that all potato chips exceed the legal limit of acrylamide by at least 39 times and some exceeded the limit by over 900 times! Acrylamide is formed when carbohydrate-rich foods are cooked at very high temperatures. So it doesn't matter whether the chips are fried or baked, even the so-called "healthier" chips contain high levels of acrylamide. A European project, known as Heat-Generated Food Toxicants (HEATOX) published in 2007, found over 800 heat induced compounds many of which are potentially cancer-causing.

The chemical Bisphenol A (BPA) can leak from baby bottles, cans and storage containers and is then absorbed into our bodies. BPA has been linked to breast cancer, prostate cancer, infertility, early puberty in girls, obesity, and attention deficit hyperactivity disorder. 93% of Americans have detectable levels of BPA in their bodies. A study was conducted in California to see if we could reduce our exposure to BPA - Food Packaging and Bisphenol A Study. BPA levels were measured in 5 families subjected to a diet of foods packaged in plastics or cans. BPA levels were measured again after the families switched to a diet of foods contained in glass and stainless steel containers. Within 3 days of switching to glass and stainless steel containers their BPA levels dropped by 60%. This study was published in the journal Environmental Health Perspectives.

BHT (Butylated Hydroxytoluene) added to cereals and breakfast bars to preserve taste, has been linked to cancers, allergies and abdominal issues.

Carrageenan is ubiquitous and found in numerous meat and dairy products, it has been linked to cancers and specifically colon cancer.

High Fructose Corn Syrup is a cheap filler added to many foods and has been linked to obesity, diabetes, metabolic syndrome and high blood pressure. The causes of obesity are diverse and complex, however, one of the causes is the overconsumption of added sugars which are very commonly found in sodas, juices, blended coffees, and fast food restaurants. Of particular concern is the use of high-fructose corn syrup (HFCS), which has increased over 1000% in consumption rates since 1967 and now accounts for almost half of the added sugar in food and beverages and is the sole caloric sweetener in soft drinks. The average US household spends approximately $850 per year on soda alone, for a total US expenditure of approximately $65 Billion per year for the entire country.

HFCS has a different biological effect in the body as compared to glucose. HFCS directly stimulates fat production and unlike glucose does not stimulate insulin secretion or leptin production, both of which are chemical signals to the brain to decrease food intake. In other words, when we consume HFCS our bodies keep on taking in more calories because there are no signals going to our brains that we have had too much. This makes HFCS the perfect substance for food companies and restaurants whose clients will over-consume without realizing they are taking in too many calories. In fact, the rapid increased consumption of HFCS has mirrored the obesity epidemic rates in the United States. [46]

The consumption of HFCS sweetened drinks is specifically associated with obesity in children. [47]

Trans Fats are found in many foods and are highly associated with heart disease.

Sodium Nitrate, found in many processed meats as a preservative, leads to heart disease and pancreatic cancer - a study conducted in 2005 showed that people who consumed processed meat had a 67% increased chance of developing pancreatic cancer. In addition, according to the Harvard School of Public Health, eating processed meats containing sodium nitrate increases the risk of developing diabetes by about 20%.

Potassium Bromate is frequently utilized in processed breads in order to create artificial volume and is known to cause cancer in lab animals in addition to kidney disease and neurological conditions.

Coloring agents (Blue 1, Blue 2, Yellow 5, and Yellow 6) present in candy, macaroni and cheese, and - are made from coal tar and are used industrially to shine floors and in head lice shampoos to kill lice - they cause cancer and behavioral problems in children.

Olestra (Olean) found in fat-free potato chips, can cause oily anal leakage and serious depletion of fat-soluble vitamins - this substance is banned in the U.K. and Canada.

Brominated vegetable oil (BVO) found in sports drinks and citrus-flavored sodas, causes hypothyroidism, autoimmune disease and cancer.

Azodicarbonamide (found in yoga mats and sneaker soles) is also present in breads, frozen dinners and boxed pasta mixes - it can cause asthma and serious lung problems. Arsenic, permitted by the FDA in chicken feed to promote growth and boost pigmentation, has been shown to cause cancer in humans.

Diphenylamine (DPA), banned by the European Food Safety Authority (EFSA), used to make apples appear fresher than they actually are, breaks down into nitrosamines which are carcinogenic.

Food companies utilize food colors to make us think we are purchasing an ingredient that is actually not in the product. For example, as pointed out by The Center in the Science for Public Interest, (CSPI), Tropicana Twister Cherry Berry contains neither berry or cherry, but the purple color comes from Red #40 which has been linked to hyperactivity and other behavioral disorders in children.

This short sighted view of nutrition and health by our government is self-defeating because we end up paying for ill health and disability in the long run. Teaching children and families about nutrition and simple cooking techniques is the best investment in our country's health.

Too much sugar is bad for health and can cause heart disease, fatty liver, obesity and all of the dire consequences of obesity. According to the American Heart Association men should consume no more than 9 teaspoons of sugar daily and women no more than 6 teaspoons. In a typical can of soda there is 20-25 teaspoons of sugar! The average person in America consumes 300 - 500 calories of added sugars daily.

The FDA does not require disclosure of added sugars so food labels can be completely misleading.

Restaurants, Fast Food Chains, and Cheap Food Everywhere

Cheap processed food prices is a major cause of obesity. The relative cost of fresh fruits and vegetables is much higher than fast food and packaged sugar-laden foods. A study that followed 5000 young adults for 20 years found cheaper prices for soda and pizza was associated with increased obesity. [41]

According to the World Health Organization (WHO) the secret to overcoming the obesity epidemic is to have an affordable supply of healthy nutrient-rich foods. There is need of cooperation between the federal government, the food industry and restaurants. [42]

The rate of obesity in the US is around 30% and continues to rise despite widespread awareness of this health-altering and potentially life-threatening problem. [43]

Obesity begins in childhood with the obesity rate in young children over 10% and in older children over 15%. The obesity rate in children continues to increase with increases in diabetes and cardiovascular diseases. Obesity rates increase as these children become adults. [44]

In 2002 the US spent $900 billion on all foods and beverages, which is the lowest cost of food per capita in the world. The highest rates of obesity and all of the medical consequences of obesity (diabetes, heart disease, dementia and early death) are seen in the poor. Nutrient-rich foods such as fresh fruits and vegetables, quality meats and fish are expensive while nutrient-poor, empty calorie foods such as depleted refined grains, sugar, saturated fats and trans-fats are cheap and readily available to lower socioeconomic groups.

(Socioeconomic determinants of health. The contribution of nutrition to inequalities in health. [45]

25% of our children drink over 26 ounces of added sugar soda daily and soda intake accounts for over 15% of our children's average caloric intake. These sugary sodas and sweetened juices are referred to as "liquid candy". American children obtain half of their daily calories from the combination of added fats and added sugars. (http://www.cspinet.org/sodapop/liquid_candy.htm Accessed January 31, 2003)

The advertising budgets of Coca-Cola and PepsiCo are approximately $3.8 billion in the US annually. (http://www.adage.com/page.cms?pageId=918.)

Soft drink companies develop advertising aimed at children in order to create lifetime brand loyalty. Complete departments and conferences are devoted to create "emotional branding for kids." Most schools in the US have multiple soda machines that sell sugary drinks to students and serve as a source of funds for the school. [48]

Americans eat on average 8 times per month at restaurants, mostly fast food. Consuming restaurant food is associated with the development of obesity. The more frequently one eats at restaurants the higher the tendency for obesity. This increasing utilization of national chain restaurants is contributing to the obesity epidemic. [49]

A study looking at data from over 12,000 participants as part of the National Health and Nutrition Examination Survey (NHANES) from the Centers for

Disease Control (CDC) found that eating at a restaurant allows for an additional 200 calories per meal from added saturated fats, sugars and sodium. This means that eating out 8-10 times per month adds 2000 calories of poor nutrition. On a yearly basis this is an additional 24,000 calories! As you can see if one continues this way year after year the insidious development of obesity can easily follow. [50]

A study published in the peer reviewed journal, Childhood Obesity, revealed that 99% of the nutritional quality of 1662 children's meals assessed utilizing the standards set in the Dietary Guidelines for Americans in 50 of the largest U.S. restaurant chains, is very poor. [51]

Over 30% of American children eat fast food every day, increasing daily calorie intake, saturated fats, sugars and carbohydrates. [52]

Another cause of concern is the significant increase in snacking among the young. [53]

A study by the Society for Nutritional Education and Behavior found that foods served at national chain restaurants are high in calories, saturated fat and sodium. The nutritional value of an average adult meal at the national chain restaurants consists of 2,020 kcal, 30 g of saturated fats, and 3,700 mg of sodium. Studies have shown that we have a poor ability to recognize energy dense (high calorie) foods and to self "downsize" our portions - this is referred to as passive overconsumption of "oversized" portions of caloric-dense foods which leads to obesity. Since there is a higher concentration of fast food restaurants in conjunction with less available quality foods in poorer neighborhoods, this effect of higher caloric intake and higher obesity rates is much more pronounced in lower socioeconomic groups. [54]

Unless the demand for healthy food choices increases, national food chain executives have very little motivation to improve their menu. [55]

We can make better choices for our health. Take the journey with us and discover and embrace our ancestors' wisdom through the Sicilian Secret Diet. It is much easier than you imagine and you will be rewarded with an enjoyable quality of life and an improved health span.

United States Department of Agriculture (USDA)

The USDA (USDA release No. 0001.14, Jan 2 2014) announced it will allow schools to serve more meat and corn. This is not the correct answer to combat the nutrition problems in American children. We need to emphasize a varied, phyto-nutrient-rich plant based diet. If we are to combat obesity and truly try to achieve wellness for our children and future adults the approach must be fundamentally changed so that we create a new culture of wellness. Children need to be taught how to optimize their nutrition, how to appreciate the soil, how to grow and prepare their own foods and introduce them to local farms. There needs to be an understanding that how we live and what we eat is fundamental to our essence as being humans.

The USDA Undersecretary for Food, Nutrition and Consumer Services, Kevin Concannon has announced that $21.6 million has been allocated to increase the amount of corn based food products for our children. This is clearly the wrong approach, and the tragedy of the obesity epidemic in this country bears this out. We need to stop this system that increases obesity and emphasizes poor nutrition.

The Physicians Health Study that included over 20,000 male physicians and a second study that included over 28,000 female patients (J Hypertens. 2008 Feb;26(2):215-22) confirmed the link between excessive meat consumption and heart disease. A mostly plant based diet is the healthier diet considering that cholesterol is found only in animal products. Meat, therefore, should be consumed in small amounts and should be from animals raised antibiotic and growth hormone free, free-range and grass-fed and finished.

We cannot make America great again if our children are not going to grow up to be healthy. [56]

Pharmaceutical Industry (Big Pharma)

I am a western medicine trained physician that believes in nutrition and life-style changes, and I also believe in treating my patients with the medication they need when they require treatment.

I am also aware that I need to carefully look at the data behind each study because of the fact that pharmaceutical companies first interest is to promote the medication they created.

Big Pharma (multinational companies that produce medicines and medical devices and their lobbying group, the Pharmaceutical Research and Manufacturers of America, PhRMA) benefits from a $1 trillion yearly pharmaceutical market. The industry contributes heavily to the Food and Drug Administration (FDA) whose mission it is to regulate the same industry that butters its bread. Big Pharma spends over $200 million yearly on lobbying expenses and contributes hundreds of millions to political campaigns.

The largest drug market in the world is in America, and 7 of the 11 largest pharmaceutical companies are headquartered in the US. Only the United States and New Zealand allow direct-to-consumer advertising of drugs. The industry spends almost $4 billion yearly on advertising drugs on TV, radio, print media and on the internet. These marketing campaigns are extremely effective resulting in sales of over $1 billion for each individual drug.

Occasionally government agencies levy fines to pharmaceutical companies for bad behavior. However, these fines are much smaller than the enormous profits earned by these companies and can be looked at as the "cost of doing business". In 2009 Pfizer, the second largest pharmaceutical company after Johnson & Johnson, faced both criminal and civil charges for promoting many of their drugs, including the cholesterol medication Lipitor, for uses that the medication was not approved for. They were never convicted, but had to pay $2.3 billion settlement and a signed five year integrity agreement with the Department of Health and Human Services. GlaxoSmithKline (GSK), the seventh largest pharmaceutical company, made the diabetes drug Avandia which resulted in over 100,000 heart attacks. GSK also paid the largest fine in pharmaceutical history of $3 billion for illegally marketing the antidepressant Paxil and the asthma drug Advair for unapproved uses. Merck & Co, the fifth largest drug company, produced Vioxx. In spite of the company's knowledge of adverse heart effects the drug was released anyway - thousands of people died of heart attacks.

Goldcare presents evidence that trials sponsored by a pharmaceutical company are four times more likely to have positive results in favor of the drug and that negative data are minimized or not published. This means that doctors may not be aware of any scientific evidence that the drug they prescribe is ineffective or harmful.

The 2007 FDA Amendment Act requires that all clinical trials with at least one site in the US, post their results on clinicaltrials.gov within one year of trial completion. Big Pharma states that the above amendment has effectively resolved the problem of negative trial results. However, a 2012 audit published in the British Medical Journal showed that at best the compliance rate was 40% and 10% for mixed industry and independent trials respectively. (BMJ. 2012;344:d7373.)

It is critical for doctors and patients to have all of the information about drugs, both positive and negative, in order to make proper informed choices.

An article published in The Journal of the American Medical Association (JAMA), "Physicians and the Pharmaceutical Industry, Is a Gift Ever Just A Gift?" (JAMA. 2000; 283(3): 373-380), reports that the drug industry spends more than $11 billion per year on promotion and marketing, and about $8-$13,000 per year on each physician. This study found that simply meeting with a drug representative resulted in increased prescribing costs, more prescriptions of newer more expensive drugs, and decreased usage of lower cost generic drugs.

The cholesterol-lowering drugs called statins when used appropriately in high risk patients have very potent cholesterol-lowering effects, are anti-inflammatory, and are proven to lower heart attack and stroke risk. However, in primary prevention (low risk patients) the data is less compelling and the side effects of muscle pain and increased blood sugar, especially in women, may not be worth the benefits of the drug.

"The Ugly Side of Statins. Systemic Appraisal of the Contemporary Un-Known Unknowns". [57, 58, 59]

Our hope is that when you engage in The Sicilian Secret Diet lifestyle you too can embark on a lifelong path to wellness with a reduced need for drugs and medical devices. My experience as Director of the Dean Ornish Heart Disease Reversal Program for Atlantic Health in New Jersey has been, that those patients who adhere to an improved lifestyle frequently reduce or eliminate the need for medications and procedures.

If we expose our genes to the optimal environment we will thrive with an abundance of good health. If, however, we expose our genes to a harmful environment of a poor diet and poor lifestyle choices we will invariably develop debilitating chronic disease. An example of this is a penguin. A penguin in the natural environment of cold and ice is happy and healthy. If, however, you place that same penguin in a hot jungle, it will get sick and die. We have evolved as hunter-gatherers, with the plants around us and if we expose our genes to the optimal environment of quality food, exercise, adequate sleep, manageable stress, and loving relationships with family and friends our genes will reward us with a long and healthful life.

Supermarkets

In a perfect world we would all shop like my aunt Esterina did in Naples, Italy. After a good night sleep she would awake at dawn and make an amazing aromatic espresso with beans that she had roasted herself. She would then set out on her daily pilgrimage to buy the groceries she would consume on that day. Lunch at my aunt Esterina's house was a big deal. She would trail blaze through open markets, climb down into cramped delis, buy meat in the marble walled butcher shop, buy tripe from waterfalls of fleshy tripe, buy fish from the fisherman's wife who ran the shop, buy mixed nuts from the family who roasted and sold nuts, and she stopped at her favorite stand to buy vegetables and fruits that would be on her table later that day. She also bought fresh flowers every day from the street flower vendor. By the time she got back home her well-worn grocery bags were packed full of nutrition ready to be prepared for the day. Packaged and prepared foods were never considered. Aunt Esterina followed the traditional way of eating that had been passed down to her from hundreds of generations that came before her.

Modern supermarkets allot little space for fresh produce. The majority of the shelves are dedicated to factory processed foods. Most packaged foods are stored in a gigantic warehouse, hundreds and sometimes thousands of miles away before actually being transported to the final destination of a supermarket. It takes weeks or months before these products reach their destination. This is one reason why processed foods need added sugar and saturated fat and salt to preserve flavor.

We have recently been informed by authors like Michael Pollan, that monoculture farming is not the best way to produce nutritionally complete foods. This is also true of the foods that are available year round. Seasonal foods from local farms are fresher, better for one's health, and also better tasting. We must eat our plants in a "rainbow of colors" in order to get the necessary phytonutrients for optimal health. If we eat the same few vegetables and fruits all year round we will inevitably lack some important nutrients.

At first glance it may appear that large supermarkets offer an infinite variety of foods. However, on closer inspection, the vast number of processed foods have very similar ingredients in different proportions. A packaged mac and cheese food concoction will be the same whether I purchase it in Chicago or in Dubai. This is because the proportions of fat, salt and sugar utilized is controlled so that the product will always taste the same.

The nutritional and obesity problem in this country and around the world will not improve unless there is a paradigm shift on how the general public views food. We have some great chefs, nutritional experts, food writers and professional foodies who understand what good food is all about. Unfortunately, this is not true for the general public. Real nutrition starts from good soil which produces plants that humans eat and that directly feed the animals we consume.

Making the right choices can dramatically improve our overall wellness. Doing the right thing for our health and the health of our family is not as difficult as it seems. Eat whole foods prepared at home, exercise moderately, avoid and reduce stress, forgive and be grateful, and connect with family and friends. We can prevent disease and reverse existing disease and enjoy our lives at the same time.

Chapter 3

YA GOTTA HAVE FRIENDS

The microbiome –your friendly bacteria

OUR BODY IS AN ECOSYSTEM with a wide variety of beneficial microorganisms living inside of us, the microbiome.

When we are born we take in the microorganism present on our mother's body and these organisms then seed our digestive tract with over 1000 species of gut bacteria. Via breastfeeding we ingest the bifidobacteria that lines our mother's mammary ducts which further adds to a healthy mix of bacteria in our guts. Children who do not have a healthy gut microbiome mix have a greater chance of developing allergies and asthma.

Typically, children born of C-section do not have a healthy mix of gut bacteria because they were not exposed to the microorganisms in the vaginal canal. In a study, a gauze was placed in the vaginal canal before the baby was delivered via C-section. Shortly after birth, this gauze was then used to rub the bacteria around the baby's mouth and skin, and these babies were shown to have a much better gut microbiome.

The Sicilian Secret Diet naturally incorporates fermented foods, yogurts and prebiotics in the form of a wide variety of good fibers that help support a healthy gut microbiome. This diet emphasizes foods such as garlic and leek which contain high levels of inulin, which is a very good prebiotic fiber that feeds the healthy bacteria in our guts. Garlic also has antibacterial properties which surprisingly selectively kills only the bad bacteria.

We have over 100 trillion bacteria on our skin, in our guts and throughout our bodies. We have about 2 pounds of bacteria in our guts. Generally, the more diverse the mix of bacteria the healthier we are and the more likely we are to lose weight and keep the weight off. There is a growing body of evidence that an unhealthy gut microbial mix leads to obesity, diabetes, heart disease, anxiety, depression, inflammatory bowel disease, liver disease, autoimmune disease and cancer.

We can cure an infectious condition called C. Difficile Enterocolitis by fecal transplants. Fecal transplants can be considered a super probiotic. A healthy person's fecal material implanted into the intestines of the infected person can be curative in most cases. Fecal transplants have also been shown to improve metabolic syndrome, insulin sensitivity and pre-diabetes, by normalizing the friendly bacterial mix.

Justin Sonnenburg, a microbiologist director of The Sonnenburg Lab at Stanford University, specializes in the intestinal microbiome research. He has stated that the human body has adapted to host the bacteria that live inside us rather than the other way around. This point of view emphasizes the importance of the symbiotic relationship with the microorganisms we share our inner environment with and the importance of a good bacterial mix for our health and well-being. In other words, we and the microorganisms that live inside us are all part of an ecosystem that includes the soil and plants that we derive nutrition from.

Recent research from the Marine Biological Laboratory (MBL) in Woods Hole, the Forsyth Institute in Cambridge and Washington University in St. Louis has shown the amazing mix of a healthy gut microbiome by using probes that light up each bacterial species with a different color. [60]

One of the largest microbiome studies ever conducted in humans was established by China-Canada Institute researchers. It evaluated the gut bacteria of 1,000 Chinese individuals (age ranges from 3 to over 100 years old). The results showed

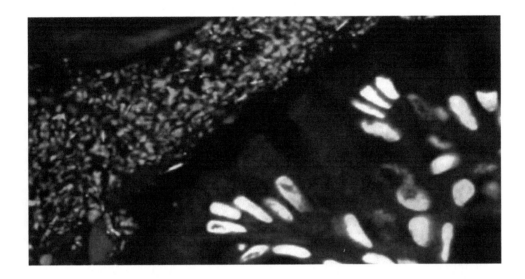

a direct correlation between the quality and mix of microbes in the intestines and the individual's health. In this study the gut microbiome of the healthy elderly group was similar to that of a healthy 30 year old. The researchers concluded that if one is able to stay active, eat well and keep a healthy mix of gut bacteria, one will experience a long and healthy life. [61]

As a cardiologist I am interested in gut health because inflammation is the key underlying factor for many degenerative diseases, including heart disease. One of the most frequent ways that inflammation starts is via a disruption of the friendly bacteria that live inside our gut. Our lifestyle choices - the quantity and quality of our food we eat, our body weight, exercise, stress, smoking, the use and abuse of certain medications such as antibiotics will continue to affect the quality, quantity and diversity of our microbiome for better or worse.

This is important because in recent years we've become more aware that an imbalance of the gut microbiome can cause low-level inflammation which can then travel from the gut to other parts of our bodies such as the heart and the brain. The microbiome can affect our brains, our behavior, our mood and mental status. It has an impact on immunity, body weight, diabetes, insulin, appetite, metabolic rate, and our propensity to develop cancer, heart disease and blocked arteries. These little guys are truly our best friends and we need to treat them well by feeding them with a good diet so that they can reward us with a healthful life.

One of the key functions of the gut is to break down food and absorb the necessary nutrients to provide for the trillions of cells that inhabit our bodies. This process separates the nutrients from waste and from the noxious particles that should pass through us and not be absorbed. A key part of the gut that protects us from these toxic substances is a lining called the epithelial layer. The fuel that sustains the epithelial layer, short-chain fatty acids, is produced by the friendly bacteria - our gut microbiome. So, anything that can negatively affect our gut microbiome can create a breakdown of the protective epithelial layer and result in what is referred to as "leaky gut syndrome" (LGS). What this means is that the gut is now malfunctioning, no longer working as a barrier between our inner body and the noxious substances and inflammation ensues.

Frequent causes of LGS are excessive alcohol intake and the SAD, which is low in fiber and high in sugar and saturated fats. Excess sugar leads to elevated insulin levels which also contributes to the inflammation process. Our body tries to fight off these invading substances by developing antibodies and other immunological responses in an effort to heal. Unfortunately when LGS is chronic the immunological response also becomes chronic resulting in food and other allergies, asthma, autism, arthritis, celiac disease, thyroid inflammation, and many other serious conditions. The solution is to heal the gut and reverse LGS.

Fortunately, simple lifestyle changes, such as the Sicilian Secret Diet, can have dramatic beneficial effects on our bacterial friends and our health. Here are some ways that the Sicilian Secret Diet Plan can help your microbiome be as healthy as possible:

- **Moderate but consistent exercise helps our friendly bacteria. In a study published in the journal GUT, Irish athletes were found to have a much better microbiome (that is, less inflammation and a more diverse gut bacteria) than the sedentary controls. In addition, exercise results in the release of beneficial chemicals such as nitric oxide, that helps improve the health of the arteries which reduces inflammation.**
- **Eat a consistent nutrient-rich, mostly plant-based diet.**
- **Meditate regularly, and consistently connect with family and friends.**
- **The healthy mix of microorganisms inside the gut will become optimal and happy and the ensuing benefits will follow.**
- **Maintaining an optimal weight helps keep our friendly bacteria healthy and in turn a healthy microbiome mix helps keep the weight in optimal ranges. There is evidence that an altered gut microbiome leads to obesity and diabetes. What appears to occur is that the gut bacterial mix changes to a type that absorbs and retains more calories from food and therefore leads to obesity. [61a]**

There is a fine balance in the symbiotic relationship between the intestinal microbiota and its mammalian host. The disruption of this fine balance contributes to the pathogenesis of many diseases. Emerging data has linked intestinal dysbiosis to several gastrointestinal diseases including inflammatory bowel disease, irritable bowel syndrome, non-alcoholic fatty liver disease, and gastrointestinal malignancy.

There is evidence that transplanting the gut microbiome from an obese individual to a lean individual will predispose that individual to obesity despite eating the same as before the transplant and vice versa. [62]

This information is important because antibiotics and hormones added to meats and dairy can disrupt the microbiome and change it into the obesity-promoting type. Antibiotics consumed early in life alter the murine colonic microbiome and contribute to adiposity.

Our ancestors have taught us that a healthy lifestyle and the consumption of quality unadulterated foods is a simple answer to a healthier microbiome. [63]

Cells in our bodies have their own internal circadian rhythm, metabolizing nutrients at different rates at different times of the day. There is evidence that our fat cells may metabolize carbohydrates better in the earlier part of the day than in the evening. Furthermore, there is evidence that the gut microbiome may interact with the cells lining the gut, and influence the amount of fat absorbed from food. This may explain why people who eat late at night or who work the night shift or who travel abroad frequently have disrupted circadian clocks and have higher rates of obesity, diabetes and heart disease. [64]

The Sicilian Secret Diet is fiber-rich, nutrient-dense and loaded with organic vegetables. As mentioned in Chapter 1 the SAD is heavy in refined sugar and low in fiber and encourages the overgrowth of "unfriendly" bacteria and other harmful microorganism such as candida which can lead to a leaky gut and uncontrolled inflammation. The Sicilian Secret Diet is a mostly plant-based diet rich with colorful phytonutrients and fiber that will help the friendly bacteria to flourish and kill the harmful microorganisms that may be living inside you. The Sicilian Secret Diet is rich in fruits, legumes, vegetables and whole grains which are a great source of fiber that enhances the life of the friendly bacteria. The amount of fiber ingested daily can influence weight, blood sugar and the gut's health. It can help the good bacteria produce a protective mucous layer which is essential for gut health, for the absorption of good nutrients and for inhibiting the absorption of noxious substances. Western diets lack in fiber creating downstream deleterious effects such as decreased friendly bacteria, increased "unfriendly" bacteria, and reduced protective mucous layer. This results in a leaky gut, widespread inflammation and metabolic diseases such as obesity, diabetes, heart disease, and cognitive decline.

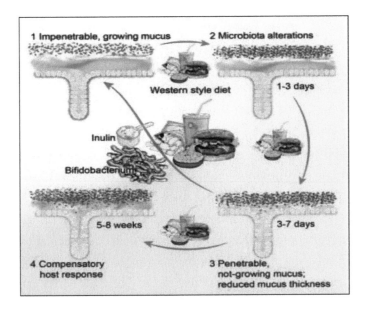

A visualization of the changes to the colon and the gut bacteria after eating a low-fiber, Western-type diet and then subsequently eating a diet supplemented with fiber. 65 Credit: Shroeder, et al.

Two recent studies found that the protective mucous layer can be lost only after 3-7 days of consuming a diet lacking in fiber and that switching to a low fiber diet resulted in a significant death rate of the friendly bacteria.

A study performed at Georgia State University found that adding the types of fiber that are a natural part of the Sicilian Secret Diet, restores the beneficial bacterial mix, reduces inflammation and improves gut health. They also found that adding healthy fiber can help reverse the metabolic syndrome. Metabolic syndrome includes a group of conditions such as obesity, high blood pressure, high blood sugar, abnormally high levels of triglycerides, and abnormally low levels of HDL cholesterol or "good" cholesterol. People with metabolic syndrome have an increased chance of developing diabetes, heart attacks and brain attacks (strokes). [66]

The Sicilian Secret Diet offers a variety of plants, fruits, whole grain cereals, tea, coffee and wine which have good concentratons of health-promoting substances called polyphenols, which include both flavonoids and non-flavonoids. Polyphenols have been shown to enhance the growth of good gut bacterial mix and simultaneously kill noxious or "bad" bacteria. In addition, studies looking at inflammation by measuring inflammatory markers in our blood (CRP levels) have shown polyphenols lower inflammation most likely by favorably affecting our friendly gut microbiome. Red wine polyphenols have been shown to reduce blood pressure, triglycerides, and cholesterol. [67]

The Sicilian Secret Diet emphasizes foods like asparagus, artichoke, root vegetables, garlic and onions which are highly nutritious and contain beneficial substances such as inulin which work as "prebiotics" - substances that help to feed and promote our friendly bacteria. Cheeses and fermented green olives, common in the Sicilian Secret Diet, work as "probiotics" and are rich in good bacteria that help maintain a healthy microbiome. [68]

Recent research supports that cruciferous vegetables like broccoli and Brussels sprouts, abundant in The Sicilian Secret Diet, protect the gut from becoming "leaky" and the resultant inflammation. These vegetables contain an organic chemical compound called indole glucosinolates, which breaks down into other compounds, including indolocarbazole (ICZ) in the stomach. ICZ binds to and activates the Aryl hydrocarbon receptor (AHR) in the intestinal lining maintaining a healthy bacterial mix, improving immunity, and strengthening the barrier function of the endothelium to keep out unwanted toxins and harmful bacteria. All of this helps to prevent the initiation of inflammation and disease associated with inflammation such as heart disease, brain aging and cancers. [69]

There's a known connection between excessive consumption of red meat and heart disease. We've always assumed this was due to the high concentration of saturated fats in red meats, however, studies now bring this connection into question. It may not be the fat in red meat that is to blame but rather other chemicals. The Cleveland Clinic's Stanley Hazen, M.D., Ph.D., published a paper in Nature Medicine describing that red meat contains elevated concentratons of chemicals such as choline and carnitine that are metabolized by gut bacteria which in turn produce trimethylamine-N-oxide, or TMAO that can cause atherosclerosis.

Avoid Toxins

We live in a world full of toxic chemicals such as phthalates that are present in fragrance products and parabens that are present in many lotions. Certain chemicals such as glyphosate may selectively kill healthy bacteria. Many synthetic fragrances, skin products and skin cleaners contain estrogen-like chemicals called xenobiotics. All these toxins can negatively affect the friendly bacteria.

Avoid as many pollutants and toxins as you possibly can. I would recommend checking the Environmental Working Group website - www.ewg.org.

Clear your head to clear out stress

As an older and hopefully wiser man, I have learned that an optimistic attitude and positive sentiments such as forgiveness, gratitude, and love has improved the quality of my life experiences but, believe it or not, it can also improve the health of your gut microbiome and help reduce inflammation.

Stress affects the friendly bacteria negatively and decreases immunity. According to researchers at Ohio State University, stress can change your gut microorganisms for the worse and can lead to the overgrowth of harmful bacteria like Clostridium. This abnormal change decreases immunity, increases inflammation, asthma, and other serious illnesses. [70]

The link between gut bacteria and anxiety has been well described in recent years. Eating the correct balance of foods, as in The Sicilian Secret Diet, helps to improve mental health by influencing the genes in the brain via a healthy gut microbiome. There is a barrier between our brains and our bodies, the blood-brain barrier, that makes it difficult for chemicals to enter our brains but friendly bacteria can easily pass through this barrier and positively influence our genes. [71]

Finally, there's even evidence that a healthy microbiome signals our brain to eat healthy foods, while a dysfunctional microbiome signals our brain to crave unhealthy foods, such as excessive carbohydrates and sugars. Interestingly, a healthy gut bacteria mix produces chemicals like serotonin that can help cope with stress. Chronic stress kills the helpful bacteria and replaces them with unfriendly bacteria creating a vicious cycle.

We may be on the verge of discovering the optimal mix of gut bacteria that could help prevent heart disease and other illnesses.

Avoid medications, especially antibiotics

Antibiotics have helped humans thrive and live through serious infections over the years and have been "miracle drugs" as far as human survival is concerned. However, overuse of antibiotics in both humans and farmed animals wreaks havoc on our friendly bacteria and results in antibiotic-resistant infections. [80]

Antibiotics administered to animals in low doses have been widely used as growth promoters in the agricultural industry since the 1950s. We believe that such sub therapeutic administration alters the population structure of the gut microbiome as well as its metabolic capabilities.

We're beginning to learn from a number of leading researchers, including from Martin Blaser, M.D. (director of NYU's Human Microbiome Program and author of Missing Microbes: How the Overuse of Antibiotics is Fueling Our Modern Plagues), that our over reliance on antibiotics can negatively affect our friendly bacteria and may lead to diseases like asthma, food allergies, diabetes, and obesity

According to the CDC, forty seven million unnecessary antibiotic prescriptions are given to patients yearly. Most infections such as colds, flu, sore throats and bronchitis are caused by viruses and not bacteria, so antibiotics are ineffective for viruses, can destroy friendly bacteria and contribute to the serious problem of antibiotic resistance. In addition, some antibiotics can cause heart problems including cardiac sudden death.

It is recommended to wait seven to 10 days before starting an antibiotic. Be wise when you speak with your doctor. Garlic, onions, fruits and vegetables are natural antivirals and antibiotics plus they offer a variety of nutrients that can help combat a common cold. [81]

Chapter 4

NICE GENES!

How you can affect the ability of your genes to do their job

"YOU CAN'T CHOOSE YOUR PARENTS," the saying goes, which means we can't choose our genes. In 1953 Watson and Crick showed the world the shape and nature of the human genetic code. We believed we were looking at the "blueprint" that determined the shape and length of our lives.

Perhaps, most importantly is the knowledge that we are not doomed to die in our fifties of a heart attack just because our fathers and grandfathers have.

Today, we've learned that our genes do play a role in our health but a relatively small one: 20 percent is the figure scientists agree on. The other 80 percent? Lifestyle. (diet, environment, habits, etc.) More earth-shifting news: what we eat, as well as how we live, meaning our social life, our satisfaction with the work we do, family connections and so on, affect the "expression" of our genes! That's right; something we have thought of as fixed—our genes and their actions on our health—is not.

The emerging fields of epigenomics and nutrigenomics are shedding light on the fact that our genes alone do not determine our fates. In other words if we are born with a gene for a certain disease we are at higher risk to develop that disease, but our lifestyle can determine if we do or do not develop the disease. For instance, people who have abnormal variants of the APOE gene are at higher risk of developing Alzheimer's disease. However, recent research has shown that adhering to a healthy lifestyle similar to the Sicilian Secret Diet, can prevent mental decline. What this means is that while we should all be adhering to a healthy lifestyle, those of us with abnormal genes need to be particularly mindful. [82]

We are entering the age of nutrigenomics, the study of the effects of nutrition on genetic expression and, in particular, the relationship between foods and disease. The compounds in certain foods have been found to increase the risk of cancer, diabetes, stroke and heart disease. Conversely, the compounds in quality foods prevent and even reverse disease. These foods are referred to as "functional foods."

Functional foods are rich in medicinal compounds that support health and longevity. These foods are *clinically proven* to prevent and treat serious disease.

How much nicer (and less expensive) it is to get your "medicine" at the grocery store rather than at the pharmacy counter!

The diverse cultures that have influenced the formation of the modern day Sicilian Secret Diet have done so over thousands of years. Trial and error over this long period of time have incorporated those foods that are best for our genes and our health. The default for our genes is to keep us living long and well because, what determines the actual outcome of our genetic potential is the environment we expose our genes to. This has been observed scientifically by the pioneering studies of Dr. Dean Ornish that showed that improving lifestyle (diet, exercise, stress reduction and improving interpersonal connectivity) can "turn off" those genes that lead to serious diseases like cancer. [83]

The Sicilian Secret Diet can help us by protecting the good genes we are born with and keep the bad ones turned off which, after all, is a gift from our parents and ancestors.

Improved lifestyle can help us live longer

The telomere is a part of our genetic code found at the end of chromosomes that protects the chromosome from breaking down. Healthy telomeres protect us from aging and dying. If we can imagine the chromosome to be a shoelace, the telomere is the plastic parts at the end of the shoelace. The longer the telomere the longer the chromosome will survive. There is scientific evidence that a healthy lifestyles lengthen the telomeres, which explains why Sicilian centenarians made it to an advanced and healthy age. [84]

Dan Buettner in The Blue Zones Solution, writes about the long-lived people of Nicoya, Costa Rica. This is one of the so-called "Blue Zone" areas of the world where people via diet and lifestyle live long and well. The telomeres of these people were studied and found to be the longest of all the groups living in Costa Rica. [85]

Nutrigenomics is the study of how food, at a molecular level, affects our genes. Everything that happens to living organisms, including humans, is a manifestation of genetic expression. If we expose our genes to a bad environment (lack of exercise, smoking, poor diet, etc.) the manifestation of our genes will be of sickness. On the other hand, if we expose our genes to a healthy environment (good food, moderate exercise, low stress, and connection to friends and family) the manifestation of our genes will be of health.

What is truly amazing is that our genes can improve for the better at any stage of our lives including in our 80s and beyond. The Lyon Diet Heart Study observed the results of a diet similar to the Sicilian Secret Diet in patients who had evidence of heart disease. Patients who followed this diet reduced further risk of heart disease by up to 70%. The results were consistent in 50 year olds and beyond! [86]

A healthy diet allows genes to express for optimal health and to protect themselves from damage to which they are constantly exposed. Food can alter DNA for the better or worse by affecting what is called single-nucleotide polymorphisms

(SNPs). Small changes in one molecule of the DNA can have dramatic health consequences. An example of how diet can interact with a SNP is the C677T polymorphism of the methylenetetrahydrofolate reductase (MTHFR) gene. Individuals positive for the MTHFR gene are less able to use the vitamin folic acid to convert homocysteine to methionine creating elevated homocysteine levels which increases the chance of developing heart disease. The Sicilian Secret Diet offers a diet ample of folate-rich vegetables such as spinach, asparagus and other green leafy vegetables that can help to override problems in unsuspecting individuals who may have SNP or DNA defect.

There is increasing evidence that genome instability, in the absence of overt exposure to genotoxicities is itself a sensitive marker of nutritional deficiency. [87]

We are in the midst of a revolution in genetics and medicine

Approximately 10 years ago it would have cost tens of millions of dollars to sequence the human genome, today this can be done for a thousand dollars and the cost is dropping on a daily basis. Since the human genome was first sequenced, we have been able to shed light on a person's predisposition for many diseases. Knowing one's risk for heart disease, cancer, depression, Alzheimer's and many others, can help one determine how aggressive to be with preventative modalities and lifestyle changes.

Epigenetics, the study of how the environment influences our genes for the better or worse, has also emerged during this past decade. Simple things, like enjoying the outdoors or the company of family and friends can also positively affect our genes. As published in the prestigious scientific journal, Proceedings of the National Academy of Science (2008;105:8369), Dr. Dean Ornish demonstrated that simple lifestyle measures such as exercise, nutrition, and stress reduction can turn off those genes that code for breast and prostate cancer.

Our genes have evolved with us over millions of years. Until very recent times it was very difficult for humans to survive. We were hunter-gatherers with very little exposure to saturated fats, sugars and salt. We went through frequent periods of famine and our genes adapted to absorb the greatest amount of nutrition from our food in order to help us survive. We were by necessity, moving all day long, exposed to the sun and vitamin D. Recently, our genes have been bombarded by the "gifts" of modern life - processed foods, added saturated fats, added sugar, added salt, low levels of exercise, stress, isolation - which has resulted in our genes expressing themselves in a negative way. Our genes are being exposed to a negative environment and the consequence is the development of chronic diseases such as arthritis, dementia, heart disease and cancers.

Genes determine whether we will be vital and energetic or fatigued and ill. Our genes' default mode is to keep us well. Most genes can be influenced by the environment to which they are exposed. The SAD includes processed foods, saturated fats, refined carbohydrates, and sugar, and because of it can influence the genes to express degenerative diseases such as heart disease, cancer and Alzheimer's. A Mediterranean diet like the Sicilian Secret Diet, rich in quality food, moderate exercise, and low stress will influence the genes to maximally code for wellness. The good news is that changing diet and lifestyle can change the course of degenerative illnesses by improving these gene expressions.

To better understand epigenetics is to realize that every cell in our body contains the same genetic material. The way a cell knows to become a heart cell, a kidney cell, a liver cell, etc., is by where it happens to be located when it is developing. In other words, the environment of the cell determines the type of cell that it will be. Similarly, queen bees are genetically identical with worker bees until they eat royal jelly which transforms them into queen bees - the royal jelly had an epigenetic effect on the bee.

We are all able to become "queen bees" by simply eating the right foods. Quality food that you will learn to utilize in The Sicilian Secret Diet is our "Royal Jelly".

The adult brain, which until recently was believed not to be able to grow or repair itself, has been shown to be able to do so if exposed to the correct environmental factors. Calorie restriction, intermittent fasting and foods like polyphenols and polyunsaturated fatty acids (PUFAs) have been shown to improve "brain plasticity", cognition, mood, anxiety, brain aging, and Alzheimer's disease. [88]

In addition, exercise works synergistically with other environmental factors to beneficially affect genes. As one adds more lifestyle changes, the benefits become not just additive but exponential with dramatic improved wellness. [89]

A healthy lifestyle can change genes for the better and these improved genes can be passed down to offspring. These positive effects can be seen for multiple generations. So, the dictum that in order to avoid heart disease one needs to pick his or her parents correctly is very true - not only from a genetic standpoint but also from a lifestyle one. [90]

Foods rich in vitamins and minerals such as folic acid, Vitamin B12, niacin, Vitamin E, retinol, and calcium are associated with a healthy DNA. High-fat diets, tobacco, and excessive exercise have been shown to damage DNA, while low-fat diets, high in cruciferous vegetables, vitamin C, and dietary fish improves the health of DNA. Foods in The Sicilian Secret Diet are a natural and rich source of all these beneficial compounds.

Diets high in riboflavin and low in folate are particularly damaging to the DNA. Excessive consumption of red meat which is high in riboflavin, excessive consumption of alcohol which can deplete folate, and poor vegetable intake, which is a rich source of folate, are bad a combination for DNA health and may help to explain the higher cancer risk seen in people that adhere to the SAD. On the other hand, The Sicilian Secret Diet offers a diet that is low in saturated fat and red meat, and is mostly plant based, which may help explain why it is associated with wellness and longevity.

Many chronic diseases such as heart disease, diabetes, obesity, dementia, Alzheimer's disease and many cancers have been determined by medical anthropologists to be "diseases of civilization." When primitive or aboriginal cultures begin to adopt a high-sugar, high-fat, "Western diet (SAD)", obesity and diabetes rates appear and increase depending on the rate that they incorporate this new way of eating. This has been well documented in the Pima Indians of Arizona and in the indigenous people of Hawaii. In both of these examples, the abandonment of the traditional plant-rich, high-fiber diet was followed by dramatic increases in the rates of obesity, diabetes and cancers. [91]

Chapter 5

ON FIRE!

Why inflammation is so important

INFLAMMATION IS A NORMAL RESPONSE to injury and infections and is essential for the healing process to begin. For instance, when we bump our leg we develop the hallmarks of inflammation - swelling, pain, and redness. This short-term inflammatory reaction is necessary to allow healing to take place. Factors such as high cholesterol, smoking, high blood pressure, nutritional deficiencies, emotional stress, lack of exercise, lack of sleep, and Western style diets cause a chronic and unremitting inflammation which in turn leads to chronic diseases such as heart disease, hypertension, cancers, dementia, Alzheimer's disease, chronic pain, obesity, ADD/ADHD, diabetes, stroke, migraine headaches, and premature aging.

The key to the longevity of Sicilian centenarians and supercentenarians may be low levels of inflammation due to lifestyle and diet.

There is scientific data that shows that inflammation can turn precancerous cells into actual cancer cells and promote metastasis (spread of cancer through-out the body). There is also evidence that depression may be caused by infections and inflammation and could be improved by reducing the inflammatory process. In addition, it is well known that inflammation in the mouth, periodontal disease, is associated with inflammation in other parts of the body and anti-inflammatory measures will also help periodontal disease.

The Western style diet or the Standard American Diet (SAD) is particularly inflammatory because it lacks important micronutrients and is rich in fat, simple sugars and salt. The SAD also causes abnormal immune responses creating allergies, food allergies, atopic dermatitis and obesity. [92]

Inflammatory foods such as red meats, processed meats and soda create an inflamed environment and stimulate the development of serious illness such as colorectal cancer. In a recent analysis researchers found that people who consume inflammatory foods are 44% more likely to develop colorectal cancer. [93]

The Sicilian Secret Diet is a natural anti-inflammatory diet rich in beneficial micronutrients, is naturally low in fat, simple sugars and salt, and promotes health in the most delicious way.

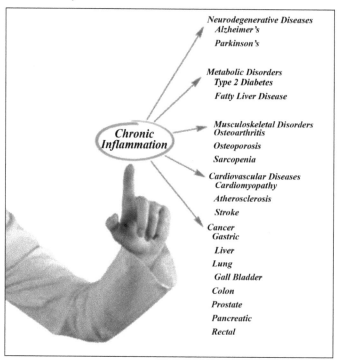

Inflammatory mechanisms caused by the brain's immune system drives the progression of Alzheimer's disease, according to new research. [94] Credit: © Dmitry/ Fotolia

Sarcopenia, or the loss of muscle mass is a problem that starts at age 40 and continues into our older years. This loss of muscle mass slows down our metabolism, can cause fall-related injuries and has a significant effect on overall health and quality of life. There is evidence that this may be due to what is referred to as "inflammaging" - in other words aging secondary to chronic inflammation. One of the markers of inflammation is called CRP, or C-Reactive Protein which stops muscles from forming proteins, so the muscles cannot repair themselves or grow as they do in a non-inflamed state.

Reducing inflammation with the Sicilian Secret Diet & Lifestyle, will help avoid the inflammation related diseases including sarcopenia. [95]

5 Quick tips to reduce inflammation:

1. **Ingest pre and probiotics that are naturally present in The Sicilian Secret Diet. It helps heal the gut, restore the optimal mix of friendly bacteria, and reduce inflammation in the heart and throughout the body.**

2. **Eat anti-inflammatory foods such as vegetables and fruits of different colors (rainbow of foods) throughout the day. The wide variety of phytonutrients, vitamins and minerals found in vegetables and fruits are readily absorbable into our systems and have powerful anti-inflammatory effects. Use Extra Virgin Olive Oil, eat nuts (especially almonds and walnuts), and fatty fish (salmon, mackerel, tuna and sardines).**

3. **Get closer to your friends and your family. Make sure you have at least one daily meaningful social interaction with a friend or family member - plan to have lunch, share a conversation. Any interaction that has depth can reduce inflammation according to recent research from the University of North Carolina at Chapel Hill.**

4. Move and stretch. Exercises daily - walking, yoga, and stretching. 15 minutes of daily exercise can reduce inflammation. Only one hour of exercise per week can reduce the onset of depression by 12%.

5. Avoid inflammatory foods such as packaged foods, restaurant foods, (frequent source of trans fats), French fries and other fried foods, sugar-sweetened beverages (soda, diet soda, and juices), red meat (burgers, steaks), processed meats (Deli meats, hot dogs, and canned meats), margarine and shortening.

Chapter 6:

TAKE CARE OF YOUR DREAMS

The importance of sleep

WE HAVE MORE LEISURE TIME than any previous post-Industrial revolution generation yet we get fewer hours of sleep per night. We've come to believe that multi-tasking proves our character (note to self: studies show multitasking is highly inefficient). We are a society descended from pioneers and immigrants, hard-driving individuals who did whatever it took to accomplish a goal, including foregoing personal care.

Sleep? That's for babies. Less hours spent sleeping means more hours to work, acquire stuff, and achieve the American dream. Right? As a matter of fact, the answer is a resounding no.

Sleep is as important to our overall health and longevity as food and exercise.

When we are sleep deprived, two important hormones that affect appetite are forced out of their natural balance: leptin (the hormone that signals we have eaten enough and feel "full") declines, and ghrelin (the hormone that triggers appetite and a desire to eat) increases. With sleep deprivation cortisol and insulin levels rise, causing more calories to be stored as fat. Growth hormone, the most important hormone for fat burning, and the repair of cells and tissue, reaches its highest level right after we fall asleep at night. Sleep deprivation makes it so the growth hormone is overridden by insulin ensuring that the fat-burning hormone that should kick in during sleep does not, and when awake the increased levels of ghrelin increase appetite.

Lack of sleep is also associated with high blood pressure, heart disease, stroke and diabetes. Also, sleep is very important for immunity - lack of sleep can lead to more frequent viral, fungal and bacterial infections.

Chronic sleep deprivation—that's anything less than 7 hours a night for adults—is linked to the onset and exacerbation of diabetes.

Studies of patients with sleep apnea, a condition that causes a cessation of breathing during sleep resulting in repeated interruptions of sleep, prove conclusively the link between insufficient sleep and heart disease and even heart attacks.

Our national lack of sleep is making us fatter and sicker and is shortening our lives.

Rubin Naiman, Ph.D., a sleep and dream specialist at the University of Arizona Center for Integrative Medicine wrote a review: "Dreamless: the silent epidemic of REM sleep loss", where he details the various factors that cause rapid eye movement (REM). Typical sleep follows a pattern that prioritizes deeper, non-REM sleep . Only later in the night and into the early morning do people experience REM sleep (dreams). Dr. Naiman believes that we are as dream-deprived as we are sleep-deprived. He sees REM/dream loss as an unrecognized public health hazard that silently contributes to chronic diseases, depression and an erosion of consciousness. [96]

Quality sleep is essential for good health. One of the commonalities that distinguishes Sicilian centenarians from non-centenarians is that they sleep well. In fact, they usually go to bed shortly after nightfall and sleep 8-9 hours nightly. In addition, they frequently take a short nap in the afternoon.

A study of centenarians from southern Italy found that centenarians go to bed early in the evening, have no problems falling asleep, wake up early in the morning, take a nap in the afternoon and do not take pills before going to bed. The quantity and quality of sleep, and the sleeping habits seem to have a significant influence on longevity. [97]

A study published in the Archives of Internal Medicine observed a group of people from a southern Mediterranean country. The researchers found that in otherwise healthy people, napping was associated with a 37% decreased chance of having coronary heart disease. [98]

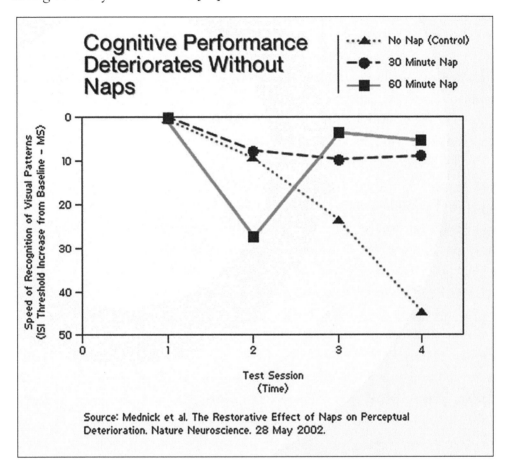

People that nap feel less pain, are less depressed and are able to put more efforts into whatever they set their mind to. A study on sleeping in Europe found that the Germans are the biggest nappers and they also happen to be one of the most innovative and productive countries in the world. Some very famous people like Leonardo Da Vinci, John F. Kennedy, Albert Einstein, Thomas Edison and Sir Winston Churchill were regular nappers.

As we strive to grow healthy and older it is important that we understand the things that protect cognitive function. There are many lifestyle factors that protect our brains as we age, such as the food we ingest, the exercise we perform, the stress we avoid, the people we interact with and the quality of our sleep.

A study performed at Harvard Medical School supports that sleeping before and after learning is critical for building memory and retaining information. Lack of sleep causes a reduction of activity in the area of the brain called the hippocampus, which is critical for the creation of memory. Even a single night of sleep deprivation can result in a significant dysfunction of the hippocampus. [100]

Sleep is critically important for optimal health. As mentioned above normal cognitive function depends on good amounts and quality of sleep. Most of memory and learning solidifies during sleep at all ages.

Sicilian centenarians maintain good mental capacity and vibrant sharp brain function. They are attentive, can make decisions and give advice.

During deep sleep, a fluid, the cerebrospinal fluid (CSF), moves more rapidly through the brain to remove toxins and waste products. Research performed by Dr. Maiken Nedergaard at the University of Rochester Medical Center, showed that when we are awake the CSF moves slowly through our brains, however, when asleep the flow of the CSF is very rapid. This is important because when awake the brain is active and accumulates significant amounts of toxins which are removed by the CSF during sleep. A special protein called beta-amyloid, which is toxic to our brains, is associated with Alzheimer's disease - this protein is also washed out during sleep. Dr. Nedergaard has termed those who do not sleep well and do not clear their brains of toxins as having "dirty brains". So, in order to "clean" your brain you need to have regular quality sleep.

Jeff Iliff a neuroscientist at Oregon Health & Science University has found that during sleep the brain cells shrink in size creating more space for the CSF to efficiently "clean" the brain. The brain represents approximately 2% of our body mass, however, it consumes 25% of our energy. This extreme metabolism results in significant production of toxins that need to be removed. This is an amazing system and is probably why sleep feels so restorative and refreshing.

Sleeping longer hours may help to better adhere to a healthy diet. Research has shown that increased sleep time results in decreased ingestion of sugar. People who get less than 7 hours of sleep nightly tend to make poor eating choices. So, getting a good night's sleep (8-9 hours) promotes health and impacts our nutrition during the day.

Sleep extension is a feasible lifestyle intervention in free-living adults who are habitually short sleepers: a potential strategy for decreasing intake of free sugars? A randomized controlled pilot study. [101]

Foods typically found in the Sicilian Mediterranean Diet, such as fish, chicken, eggs and nuts contain good amounts of tryptophan and help induce a natural good night's sleep. Tryptophan is easily converted to serotonin which facilitates slow wave sleep and rapid eye movement (REM) sleep.

Just as quality diet helps induce quality sleep, quality sleep helps maintain good eating habits. Lack of sleep is associated with overeating of fat-rich foods, simple carbohydrates, and fewer fruits and vegetables. Some researchers believe that the insomnia epidemic is related to the ongoing obesity epidemic. [127]

Fish, frequently consumed in the Sicilian Secret Diet, is associated with better sleep and higher IQ scores in children. A recent study of 541 children, 9 to 11 years old, found that children who consumed fish once weekly as compared to those who did not, scored 4.8 points higher on IQ exams and had improved overall sleep quality. [128]

Obstructive Sleep Apnea (OSA) is a sleep disorder that can generate serious consequences. People with this condition may stop breathing multiple times during the night precipitating frequent drops in blood oxygen levels resulting in a significant stress on vital organs such as the heart and brain. This is a common underdiagnosed condition affecting up to 30% of the population. Symptoms include snoring, teeth grinding, daytime sleepiness, interrupted sleep, early morning tiredness and daytime fatigue. It is frequently associated with being overweight, however it also occurs in normal weight people. It can result in heart attacks, atrial fibrillation, strokes, diabetes and obesity. It is easily diagnosed with a sleep study which can now be performed at home. The most important treatment is weight loss. A small amount of weight loss (10%) can make a big difference. Other treatments include avoiding nighttime alcohol consumption and sleeping pills; the use of a CPAP machine which forces air through the nose or mouth, dental appliances and in some cases surgery. A recent study from Johns Hopkins University School of Medicine revealed that untreated OSA can cause serious metabolic problems including high blood pressure, elevated heart rate, increased blood glucose, blood fat levels and cortisol, all of which contribute to the development of diabetes. [102]

The highest concentration of supercentenarians is found in Japan. Supercentenarians (those who live well beyond 110) tend to have very similar eating patterns - they eat freshly made whole foods and in small quantities, sleep at least 8 hours at night and nap regularly. Sicilian centenarians also have similar cultural habits and they usually eat light meals before bedtime in order to sleep well as well.

116 year old super centenarian Susannah Mushatt Jones of Brooklyn was asked in an interview by The Daily News what her secret was and she answered, "I sleep". A survey performed in the US on centenarians found that these long lived individuals place a strong emphasis on getting at least 8 hours sleep nightly.

Chapter 7

KNOW YOUR TRUE RISK

Your lifestyle calculator [81]

-**A GOOD PLACE TO START** is to calculate the risk for Heart Disease and stroke by calculating the Reynolds Risk Score: [103 and 104]

In order to complete the short questionnaire you will need to have your doctor measure the inflammation in your body by performing a blood test called High Sensitivity C-Reactive Protein (hsCRP) in addition to Total cholesterol, HDL or "good" Cholesterol and blood pressure. This risk score will help you and your doctor to assess how aggressive the lifestyle modifications need to be - weight reduction, exercise, and stress reduction.

Another good risk calculator is the American College of Cardiology and American Heart Association calculator - ACC/AHA ASCVD Calculator: [104]

Or, The Framingham Heart Study Calculators: Using Lipids. [105]

-Using BMI (Body Mass Index):

Although not a perfect indicator of risk, the Body Mass Index (BMI) is a good starting point to assess risk. It is calculated by using weight and height. An optimal BMI is between 18.5 and 25. A BMI that is too high or too low is associated with decreased health. Specifically, high BMI is associated with high blood pressure, high LDL (bad) cholesterol, Low HDL (good) cholesterol, high triglycerides and high blood glucose (sugar). A BMI greater than 30 is a measure of obesity, while a BMI between 25-29.9 shows a person to be overweight. It is possible to access the BMI calculator on the National Heart, Lung, and Blood Institute website: [106]

- **Another simple and predictive measurement for weight is to check the waist circumference. This measurement is based on the finding that when much of our fat is deposited in the mid-section rather than the hips the risk for heart disease and type 2 diabetes increases. The risk increases progressively in women when the waist circumference is greater than 35 inches and 40 inches in men. The proper way to measure waist circumference is to use a tape measure, stand, breathe out, and measure just above the hip bones.**

A good assessment tool is offered by The American Heart Association, www.heart.org.

Using their "My Life Check" calculator you can assess yourself for Life's Simple 7: [107]

- **Manage Your Blood Pressure**

- **Manage Your Blood Cholesterol**

- **Manage Your Blood Sugar**

- **Eat A Healthy Diet**

- **Maintain A Healthy Weight**

- **Keep Up Physical Activity**

- **Manage Your Smoking Status**

Body Composition

The body composition measures includes fat, protein, minerals and body water percentages. This is a great way to measure our health status and track progress as we embark on a lifestyle change program such as the Sicilian Secret Diet. Body composition can be measured with radiological studies such as x-ray absorptiometry (DXA) and CT scans or with non-radiological modalities such as Whole Body Plethysmography (Bod Pod).

Underwater/Hydrostatic Weighing, Skinfold Calipers, and Bioimpedance.

It is important to know the amount of fat in the body and also where the fat is localized. Fat distribution will contribute to the risk of developing diabetes, strokes and heart disease. One type of fat, the visceral adipose tissue (VAT) is particularly dangerous because it is found around or inside blood vessels, the heart itself and other organs and can cause inflammation, heart attacks and strokes. Increased VAT is associated with muscle loss, and can be dangerous.

A lifestyle change that is naturally anti-inflammatory such as the Sicilian Secret Diet in combination with moderate exercise is a great way to reset our body composition and to reduce the inflammatory visceral adipose tissue (VAT), the fat cells that surround our organs and blood vessels.

High Blood Pressure

New guidelines from the American College of Cardiology and the American Heart Association are as follows:

- **Normal: less than 120/80 mm Hg**

- **Elevated: Systolic (Upper number) between 120-129 and diastolic (Bottom number) between 80-89**

- **Stage 1: Systolic between 130-139 or diastolic between 80-89**

- **Stage 2: Systolic 140 and above or diastolic 90 and above**

It is important to know all of our risk factors. A simple progression from a normal blood pressure to Stage 1 doubles the risk for heart disease. The most effective way to normalize blood pressure is with lifestyle change. In many cases, medications can be avoided in the treatment of hypertension if an optimal lifestyle is adopted. The diet and lifestyle in the Sicilian Secret Diet can provide an enjoyable way of eating and living that will naturally normalize all risk factors including blood pressure.

Technology

With the help of technology it's easier than ever to keep track of our health status. We can monitor and record heart rate, blood pressure, and other vitals by touching our smartphone, checking a watch, or logging onto a laptop.

More than 100,000 health and wellness apps are available in the iTunes and Google Play stores. Some are better than others. The best exercise apps include FitStar Personal Trainer, Nike+ Training app, and Runtastic Six-Pack Abs; apps such as Fooducate, Calorie Counter, and Diet Point Weight Loss can help with diet; some of the most highly recommended apps for stress reduction are Relax and Rest Guided Meditations, Headspace, and The Worry Box. The Digital Health Scorecard app is designed to show a snapshot of health risks. It's easy to assess the health risk score by answering seven key questions and the overall health score (0-100) is calculated. The higher the score, the lower is the likelihood that we will develop diabetes, heart disease, or cancer.

"Gamification" (applying game-like elements to digital tracking devices and apps) is helpful for some when it comes to self-management, disease prevention, medication adherence, and so on. If you've ever downloaded a weight-loss app, you've probably already seen gamification in action. Typically, it includes the use of progress bars to measure success and allows users to share results with other users. Whether we share our results or simply use an app for personal accountability, these are fun tools to use that can keep motivation while acquiring new habits to improve health.

Our health care providers are using technology, too. Electronic health records (EHR) that include secure "patient portals" and allow us to view our own records, are becoming required. The information in our EHR includes results of blood tests, sleep studies, EKGs, dates of vaccinations, and other relevant information. Genomics, analysis of the function and structure of cellular DNA can also be part of digital records. Personal genomics identifies the genetic predisposition for common diseases, our carrier-status for inherited diseases, the efficacy of and potential adverse reactions of common drugs, and much more.

Telemedicine, remote monitoring and recording of certain physical functions, is being used by physicians to communicate with patients over distance, and can be instrumental when there is no possibility to see a doctor in person.

Here are some of our Favorite APPS:

Runkeeper:
- This is a great app that helps track runs, walks, and bicycling, but also helps to keep motivated.

MyFitnessPal:
- What I like about MyFitnessPal as compared to some others is that it simply tracks what we eat without trying to direct us towards a specific way of eating (i.e., low carb, low fat, etc.). It is easy to use and to set your own goals.

ShopWell:
- This app also does not try to direct the user towards a certain way of eating. You can set up your profile based on how you would like to eat, and the app will help you to buy the correct foods.

Runtastic:

- There are a myriad of sleeping apps out there, but this one truly helps to identify which factors help or hinder your ability to get a restful night's sleep.

Buddhify:

- This is a great meditation app that can be used throughout your day with over 80 short guided audio exercises.

Headspace:

- Another great meditation site that prompts you to meditate on a regular basis.

Sworkit:

- This app offers non-running fitness plans such as 7 minute workout, rump roaster, yoga for runners and others to help achieve specific fitness goals.

iTriage:

- Founded by 2 emergency medicine physicians this app helps connect patients, physicians and health plans and create personalized action plans.

WebMD:

- A mobile database with features such as a symptom checker and a pill identification tool and a medication schedule manager.

Qardio:

- Portable blood pressure and heart rate monitors.

Every Body Walk!

- Tracks walking distance, time and calories burned, and has a mapping function. It also allows users to set fitness goals.

Healthelife

- Designed to keep patients more informed by sending them push notifications and reminders. Also stores a user's health data.

Vocera

- Communication system that allows clinicians to communicate with team members. Caregivers can also use the app for emergency calls.

Esquared – esq2.com

- An Uber like app that lets one find exercise classes in their area.

FIIT – fiit.tv

- Great interactive fitness classes.

Sleep++

- Great app for tracking the quality of your sleep.

Sleep Cycle

- Tracks your sleep cycle in an effort to improve the quality of your sleep.

7 minute workout (by Wahoo Fitness)

- You can do this anywhere and no equipment is needed.

8fit

- This is a great app if you want to personalize your exercise and diet program.

Charity Miles

- A great app if you want to exercise and do good at the same time. Corporate sponsors will donate money to a nonprofit organization for every mile you complete.

Fitocracy

- An online game and social media app that utilizes gamification to help you improve your fitness.

Fitbod

- Creates a very personalized workout routine by analyzing your workout data.

C25K

- A training app that will take you from the couch to a 5K run.

Recommended Wellness Newsletters:

- Drfranklipman.com
- Mindbodygreen.com

Resources to Find Functional Medicine Physicians:

- Institute for Functional Medicine
- A4M
- Association of Accredited Naturopathic Medical Colleges

- Academy of Integrative Health & Medicine
- American College of Lifestyle Medicine

Quality Supplement and Vitamin Companies:

- Metagenics
- Thorne Research
- Xymogen
- BodyBio
- Designs for Health
- Douglas Labs
- Host Defense
- Innate Response
- Pure Encapsulations
- Integrative Therapeutics
- Life Extension
- Orthomolecular
- Researched Nutritionals
- Mountain Valley Water – Excellent bottled water

Part II
GETTING BACK ON TRACK

Chapter 8

YOU ARE WHAT YOU EAT

Sharpening your nutritional IQ

UNFORTUNATELY MOST OF THE PATIENTS that walk into my office are overweight or obese, regardless of their age, gender or socioeconomic background. During my long and rewarding career I have seen this trend growing faster and younger patients have been increasingly affected.

Most Americans are overweight and obesity is an epidemic in the U.S. and around the world.

34% of American adults and 20% of children are obese. Obesity results in devastating diseases such as diabetes, high cholesterol, heart disease, sleep apnea, cognitive dysfunction and dementia, non-alcoholic fatty liver disease, cancer and high blood pressure.

Obesity is the result of an abnormal energy balance between energy ingested through food and energy utilized through basic metabolism and physical activity.

The food environment in the U.S. has been setup for the creation of an obesity epidemic - food is cheap, ubiquitous and Americans have been served and advertised oversized portions. We are a sedentary population spending inordinate amounts of time at desks, in front of computers, watching television and riding in cars. The amount of food consumed at fast food restaurants has mirrored the rise of families in which both parents work. In spite of businesses having had to post calorie counts on New York City menus there has not been a reduction of calories purchased.

Genetically, humans are still hunter-gatherers - we still read our environment as one where the availability of food is inconsistent. Humans are just like any other animal designed to eat abundantly when food is available and to rest, unless physical activity is necessary for survival. In other words for the first time in human history we need willpower, structure and support to lower our caloric intake and to increase our physical activity.

My personal experience as a physician and health care provider has driven me to write this book, trying to provide you with the scientific evidence that supports the importance of maintaining a Mediterranean base diet. Sandra and I decided to put our expertise together and write The Sicilian Secret Diet because we recognize that people need some guidance to go back to a place where it was possible to live long and well while eating foods that taste delicious and provide good nutrition. We need to reconnect with our land, our sun, our waters and our sustainable crops.

Diseases are Reversible

This is the encouragement I want to give all my patients and all of you. We can successfully reverse inflammation and chronic diseases and it does not have to be painful.

We've all heard the expression, "you are what you eat" and now science proves it. As you learned in Chapters 1 and 2, food is the basis of our health: healthful foods promote a long life and protect us from disease while a poor diet is the root cause of disease and a shortened lifespan.

A recent study published in the medical journal The Lancet, found that participants with diabetes who lost a significant amount of weight through a combination of optimal diet and exercise were able to completely normalize the metabolic measures of diabetes. This study shows that patients who adopt a

Sicilian Secret Diet Lifestyle improve measures of quality of life. This is the key to sustaining a way of living that promotes wellness - it must make us feel better or it cannot be sustained. [108]

We have learned that our genes influence our health status based on environment, diet, and stress. In this chapter, the reader will learn how the good nutrition—minerals, vitamins, proteins, fiber—signal genes and interact with them to optimize function. It's cutting edge science that's turning previous beliefs about genetic code on its head.

What we eat also influences our mental health. Studies show that a nutritious diet and exercise can be as effective as Prozac in treating mild depression. Similarly, diet affects the brain's ability to learn and function properly. Children who are being raised on the Standard American Diet are not developing their optimal capacity to learn and think.

Centenarians in Sicily have very similar lifestyles. They eat a real Mediterranean Sicilian diet consisting of seasonal fresh fruits and vegetables, fish, whole grains, legumes and plenty of boiled greens. Their kitchens are stocked with key ingredients of the Sicilian Mediterranean diet such as fresh and sun dried tomatoes, lentils, chickpeas, pasta, onions, bay leaves, eggplant, olives, celery, basil, sardines, zucchini, carrots, rosemary, vinegar and unfiltered extra virgin olive oil. Meat is used in small quantities and usually consists of free range chickens, rabbits or grass fed lamb. There is essentially no added sugar or fat in their diets and they rarely eat between meals. They typically eat a small breakfast and supper with the largest meal at midday. The concept of a "foodie" would be laughable to these long lived people, they simply understand the correct way of eating that has been handed down to them by ancestors dating back thousands of years. They seem to put no effort into planning their meals - it is just part of their DNA. They tend to be mildly to moderately active and short naps are a common practice. A consistent theme among centenarians is the connection they have with their friends and family. The most amazing part of our research shows that opposed to America where poverty is associated with poor eating habits, in Sicily the poor manage to eat simply and well. In fact, the inhabitants of Sicily's large cities, who are wealthier, may have worse eating habits due to the influx of American style fast food and processed foods not available in the countryside.

The ability to live long and well stems from many factors but the most important one is lifestyle. It is becoming clear from recent research that even in patients who have genes that code for serious disease lifestyle factors can override these genetic predispositions. There is good scientific data that a positive lifestyle can turn "off" genes that code for cancers such as breast cancer and prostate cancer.

We are now learning that Homocysteine, an inflammatory marker, when elevated is associated with heart disease, strokes, increased chances of blood clots, Alzheimer's disease, osteoporosis, depression and breast cancer. It is of interest that the Sicilian centenarians eat foods high in folic acid, such as broccoli, beets, garlic, oranges and legumes, that naturally lower homocysteine level.

Another common inflammatory marker that is measured to assess risk of heart disease is the C-reactive Protein (CRP). CRP is one of the main inflammatory markers linked to a decreased lifespan. In a study performed by Prof. Claudio Franceschi of the University of Bologna, Italy and presented at the European Food Information Council, found that a Sicilian Style Mediterranean diet significantly reduced the levels of CRP associated with premature aging.

A landmark trial published in the New England Journal of Medicine (N Engl J Med 2013; 368:1279-1290 April 4, 2013 DOI: 10.1056/NEJMoa1200303) a Sicilian style Mediterranean diet was studied in a parallel group on a low fat diet (AHA style diet), multicenter, randomized trial. This study focused on 7447 individuals with high risk for heart disease, and the study went on for 4.8 years. The risk of combined heart attacks, stroke and death was reduced by 30%, and the risk of stroke alone was reduced 39%! A separate study on the PREDIMED (Prevención con Dieta Mediterránea) participants published in JAMA Internal Medicine, 2007, showed a significant reduction in bad cholesterol (Oxidized

LDL cholesterol) at only 3 months on the diet. In yet another study published in Diabetes Care in 2011, the Mediterranean diet in the PREDIMED participants reduced their risk of developing type 2 diabetes by 52%! The risk factors for heart disease was also assessed in the PREDIMED participants and the Sicilian style Mediterranean diet was found to have beneficial effects on blood sugar, blood pressure, cholesterol and CRP (Annals of Internal Medicine, 2006). Nuts, a common component of the Sicilian Mediterranean diet was also assessed in the PREDIMED cohort and was found to reduce the risk of dying up to an amazing 63%. BMC Medicine, 2013. [109, 110]

One of the key nutrients studied in the PREDIMED Trial was extra virgin olive oil (EVOO). EVOO is liberally utilized in the Sicilian Secret Diet. Some of the reasons why this oil is beneficial to health has come to light. A recent paper published in Biochemistry by a research team from Virginia Tech discovered that olive oil contains oleuropein which stimulates the release of insulin. Oleuropein also detoxifies a molecule called amylin that over-produces and forms harmful aggregates in diabetics and helps prevent the onset of diabetes. [111]

A study published in JAMA Internal Medicine (JAMA Intern Med. 2015;175(11):1752-1760. [doi:10.1001/jamainternmed.2015.4838) compared a Sicilian style Mediterranean diet to a low fat diet. The researcher found a significant, (over 60%) reduction in breast cancer incidence in the Sicilian style Mediterranean diet group. [112]

A Sicilian style Mediterranean Diet may help prevent blindness. Age-related macular degeneration (AMD) is a major cause of decreased vision and blindness throughout the world. In a study published in Ophthalmology. [113]

The Lyon Diet Heart Study, studied the effect of the Mediterranean diet on 605 participants who had suffered from a heart attack. One group consumed a Sicilian style Mediterranean Diet the other was given a "prudent" Western style diet. After 4 years the Sicilian Style Mediterranean Diet participants were 72% less likely to suffer a second heart attack or die from heart disease compared to those on the "prudent" Western Style diet. [114]

The endothelium is the innermost layer of cells that lines the thousands of miles of arteries in our bodies. We have recently become aware that arteries are not simply tubes that bring blood to our cells, but are active responders to the needs of the trillions of cells. In a study published in JAMA in 2004, 180 patients consumed a Sicilian style Mediterranean diet or a "prudent" low-fat diet for 2.5 years. The researchers found that the participants in the Sicilian style Mediterranean diet group lost significantly more weight, improved the function of the endothelium, reduced the inflammatory markers CRP, IL-6, IL-7, IL-18, and insulin resistance or risk of developing type 2 diabetes was reduced significantly. [115]

Another study comparing the weight loss effects of a low carbohydrate diet, versus a Sicilian style Mediterranean Diet, versus a low fat diet, found that the Sicilian style Mediterranean Diet resulted in significantly more weight loss compared with the low carb or low fat diets. [116]

It is clear from the research data that a Sicilian Style Mediterranean diet helps prevent catastrophic diseases such as heart attacks, strokes, Alzheimer's disease and Type 2 diabetes, and increases longevity.

As mentioned in chapter 4 the emerging science of nutrigenomics focuses attention on the interaction of food and genes. A study performed in Greece observed the effects of a Mediterranean diet on genes and found that this diet could override certain features of a genetic anomaly such as polymorphism. (Mol Nutr Food Res. 2016 Nov 18. doi: 10.1002/mnfr.201600558.) A study published in the September 2013 issue of Diabetes Care, showed that consuming a Sicilian style Mediterranean diet reversed the genetic risk of suffering a stroke.

There have been recent head to head studies comparing lifestyle (including a Sicilian Mediterranean Diet) versus drugs to prevent type 2 diabetes, and lifestyle was significantly more effective. As far I am concerned this is a no-brainer - I would always opt for delicious food over medications.

Foods like walnuts, well represented in the Sicilian Secret Diet, are highly nutritious and can promote health in different ways. A recent study found that adding walnuts to our diet leads to decrease in appetite and activation of the region of the brain that regulates food cravings. (Farr OM, Tuccinardi D, Upadhyay J, Oussaada SM, Mantzoros CS. Walnut consumption increases activation of the insula to highly desirable food cues: a randomized, double-blind, placebo-controlled, cross-over fMRI study. Diabetes Obes Metab. [117]

I believe that we are born with "nutritional intelligence". Our cells and our friendly microorganisms work together to signal us when to stop eating. It is possible that when we eat nutrient poor "junk" food, we tend to consume more calories because our cells are not getting the vital nutrition they need and therefore stop signaling that we are full. On the other hand, when we eat quality nutrition, our cells signal that they have had enough at a much earlier caloric load and body weight will naturally stay in the normal range. The Sicilian Secret Diet is so naturally full of powerful health promoting nutrients that you will be satisfied with smaller portions and the diet is simultaneously delicious, healthful and low in calories. The CALERIE study conducted across three sites in the U.S., showed that calorie restriction leads to healthy aging and quality longevity. This may be another reason that Sicilian centenarians are able to live quality lives well into their advanced years. [118]

What we eat and how much we eat is very important but it is not the only secret. When we eat is very important - this is the concept of chronobiology or the biology of time and our internal biological clocks. Eating seasonally and respecting the time we eat our meals are very important factors for optimal metabolism. Chronobiology takes into consideration the rhythm of life, the understanding that our hormones peak at certain times of the day, that our organs work differently at different times of the day, and that many of our senses have diurnal variations. Sleeping and napping is an integral part of optimal chronobiology. The biological changes that occur in a 24 hour period are referred to as circadian rhythms. Research shows that disruptions in circadian rhythms can lead to disease such as cancer. [119]

Recent research has shown that respecting a regular 12-13 hour fast, (for example eating dinner at 6 pm and waiting to eat breakfast at 7 am) results in reduced inflammation, diabetes and breast cancer risk and weight loss. The circadian variations are seen at the tissue level. There is evidence that our fat cells are 50% more sensitive to insulin at noon than at midnight. This may help explain the negative effects of eating late, eating in the middle of the night and the so-call "sumo" effect where sumo wrestlers gain significant weight by eating most of their calories at night. [120]

Sicilian centenarians consume the main meal of the day at midday. They typically will have a light supper, frequently consisting of steamed or boiled vegetables, a small portion of cheese and a small portion of bread. Emerging data support that the timing of feeding, especially the timing of the main meal of the day, is associated with maintenance of optimal body weight. The tissues present in the stomach, intestine, liver and pancreas have their own circadian rhythm. The timing of eating is very important for these organs so they can optimally metabolize food and eliminate waste products. Sicilian centenarians have been handed down this lifestyle rhythm by their ancestors. [121]

A useful website is: www.localharvest.org, It helps to find farmers markets, farms, and CSA's. It is always better when possible, to eat seasonally.

The food tastes better and the concentration of nutrients is at its peak. Grapes, mushrooms, squash and endives are fall foods, while citrus, kale, turnips and leeks are winter foods. The summer offers corn, peaches, tomatoes, zucchini and cucumbers. Fruits and vegetables consumed out of season are usually harvested early, refrigerated, sometimes irradiated and transported over long distances resulting in foods that are not as tasty or nutritious. On the other hand, seasonal foods have a greater chance of having been harvested locally, ripened naturally, have full flavor and are nutrient rich.

Another great way to assure the timing and source of the food we eat is to start our own garden. It can be fun, relaxing and health promoting. Get children involved. The more children learn about the importance of quality soil and the basics of gardening, the better will be their nutritional IQ. If gardening is not possible, then a Community Supported Agriculture (CSA) farm is the next best thing. Good websites to determine what is in season in your local area are: www.seasonalfoodguide.org or cuesa.org.

We have evolved together with the plants that surround us, and our cells and genes also have seasonal variations that help us digest squash better in the fall than in the summer.

The benefits of eating seasonally include better flavor, greater nutritional concentration, cheaper food because it's more abundant, and less stress on the environment because locally sourced seasonal foods require less pesticides (none is best), less genetic modification and less carbon footprint.

It feels better to be in harmony with the environment by consuming what the land has to offer.

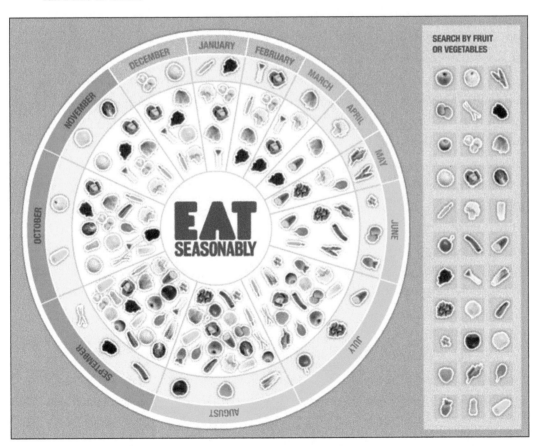

The concept of nutrient density is very important for the function of the trillions of cells that inhabit our body and this is especially true for the brain which is extremely metabolically active. Food can be "empty calories" (junk food) or nutrient dense (packed with healthful nutrients). When we consume "empty calories" our cells are still looking for the nutrients they need, making us crave more food and more calories and creating a vicious cycle of unhealthy behavior. On the other hand, when we eat nutrient dense foods, such as the Sicilian Mediterranean Diet, we need less food to meet our body's nutritional needs creating a feeling of satiety much sooner. The brain works 24/7/365 without a break. The quality of food we eat affects the brain by influencing mood and how frequently we experience a general sense of well-being. The brain requires a steady stream of good nutrients such as vitamins, minerals and antioxidants. Diets high in chemicals, sugar or added saturated fats are harmful especially to the brain. What results is brain fog, fatigue and depression.

As discussed in chapter 3, our friendly bacteria are very important for optimal health. Serotonin, a neurotransmitter that helps regulate sleep, appetite and mood, is for the most part made in the gut by our friendly bacteria. Studies have shown that taking probiotics, supplements that help maintain the good bacteria, improves mood and decreases anxiety.

Scientific publications have shown that high intake of fruit, vegetables, fish and whole grains, as found in the Sicilian Mediterranean Diet, is associated with a reduced risk of depression. [122]

A Sicilian Style Mediterranean Diet has also been shown to reduce the risk of stroke, depression, cognitive impairment, and Parkinson's Disease. [123]

There is data that confirms that an empty calorie SAD diet is associated with a smaller brain size! So, eating correctly, eating nutrient rich foods that are part of the Sicilian Mediterranean Diet can actually maintain optimal brain health. [124]

A recent study from the Memory and Aging Project (MAP), showed that a single daily serving of green leafy vegetables slows age-related decline in memory and thinking. In this study the group that ate green leafy vegetables showed a delay of an amazing 11 years of cognitive decline compared to the group who did not consume a daily serving of green leafy vegetables. Green leafy vegetables are highly emphasized in the Sicilian Diet. [125]

We need to take care of our body well. Our cells are resilient to a point, after which they will start to deteriorate, their DNA will respond by mutating and create cancer, heart disease and brain disease. By simply placing our cells and their DNA in the optimal environment we can help them thrive. Our brains are capable of functioning for 100 years and our hearts can beat 4 billion times just by eating well.

The order in which we eat our food is also very important.

Eating protein and vegetables before carbohydrates leads to a lower glycemic index and lower blood sugar levels after meals. Researchers at Cornell Weill Medical Center encouraged diabetic patients to eat protein and vegetables before eating bread and drinking orange juice and found that the blood glucose level increased only by half when compared to the group that ate carbohydrates first. [129]

Here is a simple chart that can help you conceptualize how to get organized before you actually start the Sicilian Secret Diet:

Target to achieve a more plant-based diet	Prefer and use more	Avoid and use less
Fruits and vegetables	Use more and different varieties of fruits and vegetables. Prefer seasonal products.	Inform decisions about place of production, seasonality and excessive irrigation. Avoid juices with added sugar.
Meat and dairy	Consume in moderation. Prefer plant-based proteins. Have meatless days.	Eat less red meat (less often, and smaller portions). Avoid high content of saturated fats.
Pulses	Use as protein source. Use more varieties.	Avoid salt during cooking.
Fish	Use more and different varieties. Prefer oily fish from sustainable fishing grounds or aquaculture.	Avoid fish products with high salt content, e.g. preserved fish and fish sauces.
Cereals	Prefer whole grain cereals. Use different varieties.	Avoid processed products with added sugar and salt.

The power of a healthful diet is illustrated by research that found in randomized controlled trials, an average 40% decrease in bad (LDL) cholesterol in patients placed on a whole foods plant-based diet, with moderate amounts of seeds and nuts and moderate exercise, stress reduction and social support. This is similar to the Sicilian Secret lifestyle. [131]

Randomized controlled trials have demonstrated that patients with weakened heart muscles who engage in a lifestyle change intervention show improved heart function. Patients with blocked coronary arteries (arteries that feed the heart muscle) that modify diet and lifestyle present with reduced incidence of angina (chest pain) and reduced blockage - (reversal of the abnormal process) - which continued to improve 5 years after the study was complete. Patients in the study had 2.5 fewer cardiac "events" (Heart attacks and death). These are truly remarkable results - we do not have medications or biotechnology that is this effective. What is most remarkable about these results is that the treatment (Lifestyle change) does not have any of the side effects that medications and medical devices often present, and makes patients feel better and helps them enjoy their lives. [132]

As we age our lung function declines. Foods that are regularly consumed in the Sicilian Secret Diet, such as tomatoes and apples, have been shown to slow down the natural deterioration of lung function that comes with aging. Researchers at the Johns Hopkins School of Public Health found that adults who consumed tomatoes and fresh fruit had slower decline of their age-related lung function. They also found that eating tomatoes and fresh fruit helped restore lung function in former smokers. This may be one of the reasons why people who live a healthy lifestyle are more resilient, and more able to recover from illnesses. [133]

A Word About Wine

There are numerous health benefits to the consumption of wine. First and foremost drinking wine in the company of family and friends as part of a healthful meal is a pleasurable experience.

There is evidence that regular but limited consumption of wine, especially red wine, reduces the overall risk of heart disease by lowering the "bad" LDL cholesterol. [134]

Moderate wine consumption reduces Lipoprotein (a), another independent risk factor for heart disease. [135]

People who consume wine in moderate quantities experience less heart disease and a decreased death rate from heart disease. This may be due to elevation of the "good" (HDL) cholesterol which is protective. In addition, moderate consumption of wine provides powerful beneficial polyphenols that thin the blood better than aspirin and can increases other beneficial compounds such as nitric oxide and vitamin E.

A word of caution - overindulgence has the opposite effects. Excessive wine intake can thicken the blood increasing the risk of strokes and heart attacks. [136]

Polyphenols found in red wine have been shown to help normalize insulin levels and blood sugar. Epidemiological data suggests that moderate wine consumption is associated with a reduced incidence of diabetes. [137]

Moderate wine consumption also has beneficial effects on the immune system. As discussed in the chapter on inflammation, improved immunity function lowers inflammation and lower inflammation is associated with lower infection rates and improved health. However, elevated alcohol consumption can decrease immunity and increase risk of infections and inflammation. [138]

The skin of red grapes contains a very special polyphenol called resveratrol which has an amazing beneficial effect on the heart and arteries. The very inner layer of the arteries is called the endothelial layer. Resveratrol causes an increase of nitric oxide which helps the endothelial layer dilate and become more flexible. This is very important when one considers that if we were to stretch all of our blood vessels out it would result in 100,000 miles of arteries (the earth circumference four times!) The beneficial effects of wine are multiplied when associated with a healthy diet such as the Sicilian Secret Diet. [139]

Researchers at the Gladstone Institutes have discovered that red wine can activate an anti-aging protein called SIRT1, that protects against cancer, neurodegenerative diseases, and heart disease. [140]

Over 600,000 Americans die each year from coronary artery disease. A common treatment for blockage of the arteries is coronary angioplasty, where a miniature balloon is inflated inside the blockage to open the narrowing. In addition, frequently a small mesh tube, a stent, is placed at the site of blockage to ensure that the opening stays open. A small percentage of patients treated with stents develop blockages within 6 months requiring further treatments. Researchers at Louisiana State University are coating stents with red wine antioxidants, resveratrol and quercetin, in an attempt to reduce the chances of re-blockage or restenosis.

Consumption of excessive alcohol for prolonged periods of time can have devastating negative effects on the brain, liver and heart. However, researchers at the University of Rochester Medical Center have found that low regular alcohol consumption reduces brain inflammation and helps the brain clear away toxins, including those associated with Alzheimer's disease. The brain utilizes a system of toxin drainage called the glymphatic system, which is more active when we sleep or exercise. Low level alcohol ingestion (1-2 glasses of red wine daily) may actually stimulate the glymphatic system to work better, and in turn reduce brain inflammation. [141]

A Word About Fiber

Fiber is at the top of the list of beneficial nutrients missing from a Western SAD diet. Diets high in processed foods, high in animal protein, high in added fats, salt and sugar lack quality fiber needed for optimal wellness. The Sicilian Secret Diet offers an easy and enjoyable way to incorporate the beneficial fiber needed. Americans on average consume half of the fiber recommended by the

US Food and Nutrition Board - 21-25 grams/day for women and 30-38-grams/day for men. [142]

Research data reveals that increasing fiber intake by 7 grams/day reduces the risk of a "Brain Attack" or stroke by 7%! Fruits and vegetables are a big part of the Sicilian Secret Diet. Adding just one fruit and one serving of vegetables per day will increase the daily fiber intake by over 7 grams per day. [143]

A Word About Coffee

Coffee consumption has been associated with lower risk of heart disease, diabetes and strokes.

According to a recent meta-analysis study, (a review of all of the important scientific literature on a subject), published in the British Medical Journal, drinking 2-4 cups of coffee daily is linked to a longer life. The researchers reviewed over 200 studies and found that drinking coffee reduces the risk of heart disease, cancers, diabetes, liver disease, dementia and increases overall lifespan. Coffee drinking also seems to help prevent Parkinson's disease, Alzheimer's disease and depression. [144]

A recent study also has shown that coffee can help improve the function of the mitochondria (the energy producing part found in each of the trillions of cells in our bodies) and this in turn helps protect heart cells from damage. [145]

There is evidence that coffee not only helps to enhance physical performance, but also may enhance mental performance. A study performed at The Stevens Institute of Technology found that by simply smelling coffee students performed better on a GMAT algebra test. [146]

Chapter 9

EXERCISE

It's feasible, even for you!

WOULDN'T IT BE NICE IF we could identify a simple, affordable, and pleasant form of exercise that could improve our health and extend our life? We have: it's walking. That's right, the simple act of standing up and moving, putting one foot in front of the other, will improve health, regulate weight, preserve mental sharpness, and increase longevity. No gym membership required.

A recent study published in the European Journal of Preventive Cardiology found that simply standing instead of sitting prevents weight gain and can result in weight loss. Avoid sitting for more than 30 minutes at a time then stand or walk for 5-10 minutes. A standing desk is a great way to avoid prolonged sitting while at work. [147]

Walking, scientists have discovered, is the most natural anti-inflammatory activity we can engage in. Inflammation is a mark of disease and of the environment that sets the stage for disease. Specific foods have anti-inflammatory properties and we want to include them in our diet, but the health benefits of walking are so significant that it needs to be part of our daily routine.

"Sitting is the new smoking", is an expression that has been coined to bring home the deleterious effects of our sedentary lives. Sitting for prolonged periods of time has been linked to heart disease, obesity, and diabetes. Walking is the antidote.

Walking can cure what ails you. Study after study shows that walking can help improve symptoms of mild depression and anxiety. Walking staves off osteoarthritis, atherosclerosis, dementia and other debilitating conditions and can reverse disease that has already started. A walking regimen helps ensure success when quitting smoking.

Sicilians walk at least three times a day. Walking to do errands, grocery shopping or meeting a friend in the town square are everyday customs. A walk after lunch or after dinner, to "digest" and enjoy the outdoors is as ingrained in the culture as starting the day with a steaming cup of espresso.

A study published in JAMA Internal Medicine in 2015 assessed 661,000 adults' exercise habits over 14 years. They found that people at highest risk for dying were those who were inactive. People who lived the longest were those who performed the exercise equivalent of walking one hour daily (40% less likely to die as compared to the sedentary folks). This correlates well with the physical activity of the typical Sicilian centenarian who performs mild to moderate physical activity during the day. [148]

A recent study from the Netherlands revealed that moderate physical activity is associated with reduced incidence of heart disease. Elderly people who performed low intensity exercise such as walking, gardening, cooking and housework showed a significant reduction of serious heart disease. [149]

The University of San Diego School of Medicine followed 6000 women ages 65 to 99 for 4.5 years. Women who performed light physical activity for 30 minutes daily lowered the risk of dying by 12% and those who performed an additional 30 minutes of exercise daily lowered their risk of dying by any cause by 39%! [150]

The Faculty of Sport and Health Sciences at the University of Jyvaskyla performed a four year study that shows how reductions in daily step count correlates with weight gain and increased body mass index (BMI). Study participants that increased step count by 2000 steps daily maintained their BMI, while those participants whose step counts went down increased their BMI. The recommended daily step count for adults is 10,000 daily. [151]

Another study performed in Australia examined 200,000 Australian adults and confirmed that simple moderate exercise such as walking reduced the risk of dying earlier and that occasional vigorous exercise could add an additional 9% benefit. [152]

Physical activity lowers blood pressure and rates of heart attacks, reduces inflammation, improves metabolism, depression and the overall sense of well-being. The belief that we need to exercise vigorously or run marathons in order to be healthy is far from the truth. A recent article analyzing 22 studies of 320,000 adults, shows that moderate exercise such as walking or gardening is associated with lower rates of heart attacks, strokes, and death from all causes. [153]

Studies have shown that intermittent low-intensity standing or movements throughout the day may be as effective as structured exercise for disease prevention and general well-being. The deleterious effects of prolonged sitting is most likely due to the fact that inactive muscle requires less blood glucose increasing the risk of developing diabetes. Sitting decreases blood flow which facilitates plaque buildup resulting in increased risk of heart attacks and strokes.

Sitting may "trick" our bodies into thinking that our body weight is less than it actually is. Researchers at the University of Gothenburg, Sweden have found evidence of an internal body weight sensing system. It is not clear yet how this sensing system works, however, when we stand our lower extremities send signals to the brain to adjust our food intake to maintain steady weight. This mechanism may help regulate body fat. When we are up on our feet and active, the body will more accurately signal the brain to mobilize fat. [154]

Just like food, exercise can affect our genes. A study published in the journal Epigenetics, (the Karolinska Institute in Stockholm Sweden) observed volunteers who exercised on a stationary bicycle using only one leg for three months. Multiple medical tests were performed including muscle biopsies before and after the exercise protocol both in the exercised leg and in the not exercised one. What they discovered was fascinating, the genes in the exercised leg changed in thousands of sites as compared to the unexercised leg. The genetic changes observed have a positive effect on muscle metabolism, the way the muscle responds to insulin, and the amount of inflammation in the muscle. None of these changes occurred in the unexercised leg.

Exercise can affect and change our genes for the better. [155]

Positive DNA Changes can happen very quickly, after exercising for 20 minutes. This occurs by a process called methylation. Chemicals called methyl groups attach to DNA and turn off the DNA ability to activate certain genes. When the methyl groups detach the genes are activated. Our cells are constantly regulating our genes through this methylation process. Research at the Karolinska Institute in Sweden, performed muscle biopsies on sedentary volunteers before and after 20 minutes of exercise. They found that after 20 minutes of exercise the DNA was turned on allowing the muscle to produce more enzymes and nutrients needed for an activity. In other words, the DNA is adapting to allow for more efficient muscular activity. They also found that the more the activity is vigorous the more the DNA is turned on. [156]

Exercise can improve the anatomy of our brain.

Sicilians love to dance and a recent study showed that people who engage in regular dancing grow the part of the brain called the hippocampus, critical for memory. In addition, these people showed improved balance.

Regular exercise, especially dancing, can prevent cognitive decline associated with aging. [157]

Exercise can help prevent dementia and slow the memory loss that occurs with aging. Over 5 million Americans are currently diagnosed with Alzheimer's disease, a devastating disease and the sixth leading cause of death in the United States. The number of people who will develop Alzheimer's disease is expected to triple by 2050. There is no effective treatment. A recent report from the American Geriatrics Society found, however, that older adults who performed aerobic exercise had improved brain function. This is true for people who are at risk for developing Alzheimer's disease and those who have the disease. The benefits of moderate exercise can increase both the quality and the length of our life. [158]

The American Academy of Neurology published guidelines in the journal Neurology (Dec 27, 2017) for exercise that can help memory in patients with mild cognitive impairment. The Academy recommends mild to moderate exercise for about 150 minutes weekly.

5925 women aged greater than 65 were followed for 8 years. The women who walked more had significantly less brain function deterioration than those who did not exercise. The researchers concluded that physical activity such as walking prevents cognitive decline. [159]

Mild but consistent exercise is similar to the regular low level activities that Sicilian centenarians have been performing for centuries

During Exercise hormones and other biochemicals are released into the body. Many hormones and biochemicals such as Insulin, Glucagon, cortisol, testosterone, prolactin, insulin-like growth factor, growth hormone (GH), thyroid stimulating hormone (TSH), luteinizing hormone (LH), follicle stimulating hormone (FSH), epinephrine and norepinephrine, brain-derived neurotrophic factor (BDNF), Irisin, Peptide YY, Endorphins and Interleukin-6 are released with exercise. Which hormones and the amount of hormone released varies with the type and degree of exercise performed. Some hormones, like cortisol, go down during the initial phases of exercise and then rise with continued exercise. Exercise is the most powerful stimulus for the release of growth hormone (GH), which is sometimes referred to as the "repair" hormone. GH helps endurance by stimulating the release of free fatty acids needed for energy.

This output of hormones during exercise is part of a complex web that works in concert to alter the DNA expression in order to improve functional efficiency. These hormones affect the nucleus of the cell, the cell membrane and the nervous system. The various effects of these hormones are the following:

- **Insulin - carbohydrate and fat metabolism**

- **Glycogen - helps release free fatty acids and stored glucose for energy**

- Cortisol - released during prolonged exercise, and helps break down molecules for energy.

- Epinephrine and Norepinephrine - Epinephrine or adrenaline increases blood sugar to improve energy and to facilitate more blood flow to muscles during exercise.

- Testosterone - important for both men and women for the repair and growth of skeletal muscles.

- Human Growth Hormone (HGH) - important for muscle growth and repair. HGH is released only during REM sleep or high-intensity exercise.

- Insulin-Like Growth Factor (IGF 1) - similar structure to insulin but has actions similar to GH chelping repair and promote growth of skeletal muscles.

- Brain-Derived Neurotrophic Factor (BDNF) - High-intensity exercise in addition to releasing HGH and IGF 1 releases BDNF which helps create new brain cells and improves cognitive function.

- Irisin - stimulates fat cells to burn energy. It also appears to convert white fat cells into brown fat cells which are more metabolically active and associated with reduced risk of obesity and diabetes.

- Peptide YY - a gut hormone released by gastrointestinal tract cells to influence the brain to reduce appetite. (Ann NY Acad Sci. 2003 Jun; 994:162-8.). Exercise also stimulates the release of peptide YY, possibly reducing hunger after exercise.

- Endorphins - neurotransmitters originating in the pituitary gland and in other parts of the nervous system. They work as opioid analgesic allowing athletes to feel less plain and accounting for the so-called "runner's high".

THE SICILIAN SECRET DIET PLAN

Other activities and foods that stimulate endorphin release are acupuncture, meditation, capsaicin (Chili peppers), chocolate, ginseng, laughing, sex, lavender, listening to music and massage therapy. Endorphins may also play a role in decreasing the sense of fatigue during exercise. [138]

Interleukin -6 (IL-6) - IL-6 is a cytokine and is released during times of stress such as trauma, burns and infections. IL-6 has both proinflammatory and anti-inflammatory properties. Of all the cytokines IL-6 is produced in large amounts during exercise. It has growth factor properties and helps the musculoskeletal system to recover and adapt to exercise. [160]

The outpouring of hormones, the decrease in inflammation, the increase in metabolic rate, the decreased risk of chronic disease, improved brain function, and improved genetics, are just some of the many benefits of exercise.

In 1909, Edward Payson Weston, 70 years old at the time, walked from New York City to San Francisco in 105 days. Mr. Weston set the groundwork for the elderly to exercise. Prior to that people believed that exercise for older adults was not beneficial and possibly deleterious. We now know, thanks to Mr. Weston and thousands of pioneers after him, that exercise is essential for optimal health.

Researchers at Western University, London, Canada have shown that a 10-minute, one-time burst of exercise, can have immediate effects on focus and brain power. This means that before engaging in a mentally demanding activity such as taking a test, doing your taxes, giving a speech or having an important meeting, getting 10 minutes of vigorous exercise may help to be more focused and alert. [161]

The release of hormones, endorphins and neurotransmitters such as norepinephrine improves mental status. The American Psychological Association states that exercise is a beneficial antidepressant both immediately and in the long term. They also state that all forms of exercise, including walking, are effective antidepressant measures. [162]

Other benefits of walking:

- **Reduced osteoporosis and reduced risk of hip fractures [163]**
- **Longer life [164]**
- **Reduced Intra-Abdominal Fat [165]**
- **Weight Loss**
- **Improved Sleep**

Walking is the "first step" to improved health. Walking can be done at all ages, is low impact and has a very low risk of injury. The goal for walking should be 150 minutes weekly which is easily doable or 75 minutes of intense exercise per week. Walk alone, with your partner, family, friends, with your dog, listening to music or a book, or simply listening to nature. Walking is the most natural way to prevent heart disease, lower blood pressure, cholesterol, manage weight, increase good (HDL) cholesterol, decrease triglycerides, improve sleep and improve sex life.

Chapter 10

STRESS REDUCTION AND RELAXATION

Yes, it matters

UNDER STRESS THE BODY PRODUCES cortisol—a hormone that has helped humans survive life-threatening situations. But when the stress is chronic cortisol is released for extended periods of times weakening the immune system and setting inflammation. This creates the stage for the development of chronic disease.

Studies show that chronic stress and poor coping skills contribute to arterial plaque, which is linked to heart attacks, osteoporosis, dementia and behavioral health problems such as depression and aggression.

There is a growing body of scientific evidence that positive emotions such as gratefulness, forgiveness and love increase the production of beneficial chemicals such as serotonin capable of decreasing inflammation, increasing sense of well-being and improving the telomeres, resulting in the DNA living longer. Anger, resentment and sadness, on the other hand, increase the release of stress hormones which in turn increase inflammation, cause DNA to die off sooner and can lead to a 6-fold increase in the risk of heart attack. Anger can also increase the risk of strokes and lung disease.

Negative emotions decrease immunity and increase the risk of infection, asthma, diabetes, stomach ulcers, ulcerative colitis, cancers and atherosclerosis. [166]

According to a study published in the Journal of the American Medical Association (JAMA) up to 80% of visits to a primary care doctor may be related to stress, however, only 3% receive appropriate stress reduction counseling. This may be because our medical system does allow enough time for each patient visit. [167]

A research team at Carnegie Mellon University, found chronic stress causes the inflammation regulating hormone, cortisol, to become less effective. Since one of the functions of cortisol is to reduce inflammation, a less effective cortisol results in increased inflammation and the diseases associated with inflammation. [168]

Chronic stress and anxiety frequently lead to depression which has been linked to increased heart disease risk. UCSF Medical School. [148]

The Heart and Soul Study performed by researchers at UCSF enrolled 1024 patients and followed them for over 15 years. They found that depression was associated with a 50% greater risk of cardiovascular diseases - heart attacks, heart failure, stroke and death. [169]

Stress, anxiety and depression are associated with elevated inflammatory markers (Interleukin-6, Tumor Necrosis Factor alpha, and C-Reactive Protein, and others) which promote and prolong inflammation. The good news is that stress reduction modalities, such as exercise, meditation and sleep, can reverse the process.

A 2-question test developed by Mary A. Whooley at UCSF is a simple way to screen for possible depression.

1. During the past month, have you often been bothered by feeling down, depressed or hopeless?	☐ Yes	☐ No
2. During the past month, have you often been bothered by little interest or pleasure in doing things?	☐ Yes	☐ No

"Yes" to one (or both) questions	= positive test (requires further evaluation)
"No" to both questions	= negative test (not depressed)

Emotional stress such as depression, anger, hostility and anxiety can increase free radicals in our body.

The very basic function of the food we eat is to give energy to the powerhouse of the cell - the mitochondria. The purpose of breathing is to bring oxygen to our cells and mitochondria. These two processes allow the mitochondria to use glucose, fatty acids and oxygen to create adenosine triphosphate (ATP) molecules, which are the energy molecules that maintain life. This process produces waste molecules, called free radicals, that have to be eliminated. Sometimes these free radicals can be useful because they can kill harmful bacteria behaving as a sort of natural antibiotic. But in larger quantities free radicals can causes damage to mito-chondria, and damaged mitochondria means less energy. Free radical damage is one of the causes of premature aging and diseases associated with premature aging such as heart disease, brain disease, early cognitive impairment, cataracts, loss of eyesight, and cancers. Antioxidants such as vitamin C, vitamin E and enzymes produced in our bodies such as superoxide dismutase (SOD), catalase, and glutathione peroxidase help to counteract the deleterious effects of free radicals.

There are many studies that confirm that stress such as depression, social isolation, anger, hostility, and anxiety can negatively affect DNA and speed up the aging process. In other words, stress can make one age faster. A study performed at Brigham and Women's Hospital in Boston, found that chronic stress is asso-ciated with shorter telomere length. Remember - the longer the telomere, the longer the DNA lives and the longer we live. [170]

Another study found that a person's lifetime exposure to stress and depression is proportionally related to telomere shortening – [171]

Other hormones that are affected by chronic stress include:

- **Gonadotropins**
- **Testosterone**
- **Estrogen**
- **Thyroid Hormones**

- **Vasopressin**
- **Growth Hormone**
- **Prolactin**
- **Insulin**

Disease caused by hormone disrupted by chronic stress:

- **Hyperthyroidism**
- **Diabetes**
- **Menstrual irregularities**
- **Decreased Sperm Motility**
- **Infertility**
- **Psychosocial dwarfism**
- **Obesity [172]**

Acute and chronic stress can have devastating effects on the heart. It is well documented that sudden and acute stress, such as earthquakes, the terrorist attacks of 9/11, or terrible news like the death of a child or loved one can trigger a heart attack. There is a condition called "broken heart syndrome" which results from severe and acute stress, and can result in severe sometimes life-threatening heart attacks without the presence of a blocked heart artery.

Chronic stress such as job stress, marital unhappiness, and the burden of being a caregiver can result in heart disease. The stress itself is damaging to the heart, but chronic stress can also cause unhealthy behavior such as smoking and over-eating of "junk" foods. In addition, chronic stress results in lack of motivation, reduced exercise, and insomnia increasing the risk of high blood pressure, heart attacks, abnormal heart beats, chest pain or shortness of breath. Employees who experience work-related stress and individuals who are socially isolated have an increased risk of a first heart attack. In those people who already have established heart disease, acute and chronic stress can cause recurrent problems and even death. [173]

Stress can also result in the acute release of high levels of hormones and neurotransmitters. In a study looking at doctors in training who were engaged in public speaking found significant spikes in plasma epinephrine levels during their speech. [174]

There is evidence that discrimination is a serious cause of stress and can result in heart disease. In a study looking into this, those individuals who perceived more discrimination had significantly larger increases in diastolic blood pressure. [175]

In order to manage stress we first have to recognize that we are stressed. Fatigue, low energy, irritability, decreased sex drive, binge eating are some of the symptoms of stress.

The causes of stress are multiple and can be aggravated by poor lifestyle choices such as lack of sleep, lack of exercise, isolation and poor nutrition.

Writing down the causes of stress, talking with a family member, partner, friend or therapist is a good way to identify the problems and start finding appropriate solutions.

Keeping a sleep diary, starting a sleep hygiene routine, meditation and exercise are helpful steps to reduce stress.

When we are stressed we feel overwhelmed and we avoid making changes because changes feel like adding more work to the heavy load we are already carrying.

Stress often comes from excessive worries. Anticipate that good things can happen today instead of anticipating bad or catastrophic. Look for the small positive experiences we all have every day and make note of them, a child's laugh, an act of kindness, a sunny day, the smell of rain…

Small changes are doable especially if we ask for help. Asking for help is always a sign of strength and never of weakness.

Sleep is the most important part of our day.

Make sure there are no medical reasons for poor sleep (Sleep apnea, thyroid disease, restless leg syndrome, etc.)

Create a bedtime ritual that is always the same. Avoid electronics one hour before bed. Avoid alcohol, nicotine and any other stimulating substances before bedtime. Keep your bedroom dark and cool. A hot bath with Epsom salts and lavender oils, stretching, a walk with the dog, and meditation are best bed time practices for a more restful sleep.

Exercise and good nutrition are as important as sleep for stress reduction.

Move your body throughout the day however you choose to. Make eye contact and smile every time you meet someone especially the people you love. Remember the good things that have happened to you and smile and laugh. Hold hands, hug, make love, it releases endorphins, oxytocin, serotonin and dopamine for great stress reduction.

Learn how to breathe to reduce stress. Breath is life. There are several good and accessible apps to guide you through breathing exercises, choose the ones that match your style.

Chapter 11

DOABLE DETOXIFICATION

The liver–heart connection

OUR BODY IS AN AMAZING machine, capable of converting food to energy, fighting off diseases, and healing from injury. It has a system that protects us from an array of poisons: the liver and its detoxification system. The liver is our largest organ and it plays a quiet but vital role in managing our health. It metabolizes protein and fat, stores glucose for energy, produces bile for digestion, filters toxins separating them from the bloodstream so they can be eliminated through sweat, urine, and bowels.

Today our livers are overburdened by the number of toxins present in our environment and diet. Our foods have more additives than ever (many of which are untested), and we are exposed to known carcinogens in food packaging as well as in the grass we walk on, the water we drink, and the air we breathe. This over-exposure to toxins is increasing the incidence of heart disease and cancer.

Fortunately, diet and lifestyle are the most effective tools to support the liver and that is why it is so important to buy organically-raised produce and meats whenever we can. Certain foods, which are an integral part of The Sicilian Secret Diet, including onion, garlic, artichokes, beets, and cruciferous vegetables promote detoxification and strengthen the liver, so be sure to make them a regular part of your diet. Herbs and spices such as rosemary, oregano, turmeric and other staples of the Sicilian diet are high in Sulphur and glutathione, compounds that help the liver do its job. Some Supplements can help too such as green tea extract, milk thistle, and certain seaweed extracts. Sleep has innumerable benefits, one of which is supporting natural detoxification.

The liver and gut work hand in hand to remove unwanted toxic substances from our bodies. The blood flow from the gut passes through the liver for removal of unwanted chemicals and proteins. Gut bacteria are closely related to liver health. Gut bacteria produce ethanol, ammonia and acetaldehyde and too much of these chemicals can cause liver disease. This is one of the reasons that an optimal mix of friendly bacteria inside of us is so important.

Liver health is necessary for optimal wellness. The liver is an amazing organ that knows what is good for you and what is not. It works as a nutritional warehouse and factory by combining amino acids into proteins and by storing glucose into glycogen to be released during physical activity. The liver stores other vital nutrients such as Vitamin A, D, K, B12, Folic Acid and makes blood clotting factors. In addition, it produces bile, stored in the gallbladder, helpful for the digestion of fatty foods. It also acts as a filter removing microorganisms such as bacteria, fungi, viruses and parasites from the bloodstream.

Detoxification has become another buzz word in the quest for quick answers to our nutritional woes. Commercial detox diets don't work, are not necessary and can be counterproductive by adding to the toxic load. Long term fasts can lead to muscle breakdown and nutritional deficiencies and can induce headaches, fatigue, irritability, rashes and pain. Our body has a natural sophisticated ability to eliminate most toxins as long as we reduce the toxin burden and support our natural detox system with good food.

A Study spearheaded by the Environmental Working Group (EWG) in collaboration with Commonweal, tested umbilical cord blood for toxins and found over 280 industrial chemicals including pesticides, wastes from burning coal, gasoline and garbage, many of these toxins are cancer-promoting and toxic for the nervous system.

Stress is another source of toxicity that works by increasing stress hormones and disrupting sleep which further inhibits our ability to detoxify the brain.

The Sicilian Secret Diet and lifestyle promotes natural detoxification by offering foods low in high fat foods and simple sugars, limiting portion sizes and providing a wide variety of fruits and vegetables. This may be yet another reason why there are so many clusters of populations that live to be 100 years and older throughout Sicily.

Glutathione [176]

Glutathione is a substance composed of three amino acids (tripeptide) - cysteine, glycine, and glutamic acid. Glutathione has many important cellular functions. It is a powerful antioxidant, helps regenerate vitamin C and E, helps the first and second phases of the liver detoxification process, helps get rid of mercury from cells and the brain, helps regulate cell replication and cell death, and is critically important for mitochondrial function. Chronic exposure to alcohol and heavy metals such as cadmium can significantly lower glutathione levels. The amount of glutathione at the cellular level correlate directly with longevity.

Low levels of glutathione are associated with the following diseases:

- **Brain Diseases (Alzheimer's, Parkinson's, Huntington's, Amyotrophic Lateral Sclerosis (ALS))**

- **Lung Disease (COPD, Asthma)**

- **Immune Disease (HIV, autoimmune disease)**

- **Heart Disease (High Blood Pressure, heart attacks, Elevated "bad" cholesterol (LDL))**

- **Chronic Age-Related Diseases (Cataracts, Macular Degeneration, Hearing Loss, and Glaucoma)Liver Disease, Cystic Fibrosis, Accelerated Aging**

The best way to maintain good levels of glutathione is to avoid exposure to toxins, to limit the consumption of alcohol, to consume less animal fat and more organic plants. Oral glutathione supplement is not well absorbed and does not result in significantly increased levels.

Alpha Lipoic Acid, N-Acetyl Cysteine (NAC), or SAMe are helpful supplements that increase glutathione levels. The best is NAC, because it supplies cysteine which is a key component of glutathione production. Foods that increase glutathione production are alcohol-free beer (can raise the cellular level of glutathione 29%!), and almonds. People who meditate have 20% higher levels of glutathione as compared to non-meditators.

Fish

Multiple studies have shown that eating fish protects the brain from dementia. However, as the seas and oceans become more polluted the fear of mercury in fish has risen, especially the fear that mercury could cause Alzheimer's disease. Dr. Martha Clare Morris and her team from Rush University are prominent Alzheimer's disease researchers. They studied the donated brains of 286 individuals who had completed 5 years of food journals. The researchers wanted to study the effects of mercury on the brain and the protective effects of omega 3 fatty acids from fish, plants, or supplements. They did find that higher fish consumption was associated to higher mercury in the brains at autopsy, however, mercury levels in the brain did not correlate with brain damage. Eating fish once a week correlates with significantly less Alzheimer's changes in the brains of people with the Alzheimer's gene. Regular consumption of plant-based omega 3s from walnuts, flaxseed and chia seeds protects from strokes but fish oil supplements offered no protection. This study shows that moderate levels of mercury does not cause brain damage.

A good way to reduce toxic burden is sauna bathing, and specifically infrared sauna. A study undertaken in Finland, The Kuopio Ischaemic Heart Disease

Risk Factor Study (KIHD), involved 1,621 middle-aged men. Men with a sauna frequency of 2-3 times a week reduced the risk of high blood pressure by 24%, while men who had a sauna 4-7 times per week lowered the risk of developing high blood pressure by 46%. Sauna bathing helps improve the function of the inner lining of the blood vessels, the endothelial layer of cells, and eliminates fluid and toxins via sweating. In addition, sauna bathing relaxes the body and mind which further reduces the toxic burden of stress hormones. [177]

The Sicilian Diet lifestyle, which incorporates reduced exposure to toxins, a clean plant-based low animal fat diet, exercise and meditation, naturally and easily helps boost the cells concentration of important health promoting chemicals such as glutathione.

Chapter 12

IT'S ALL ABOUT NEIGHBORHOOD

The importance of your community

OUR SOCIAL CONNECTIONS ARE THE foundation of what is referred to as the "Social Contagion Theory", in which attitudes and behaviors (good or bad) are spread within a group by imitation and conformity. By learning how to strengthen our positive social network (and depart from the negative ones) we engage in "the dynamic spread of happiness".

Social relationships are very important for overall health. People who have low quantity or low quality social relationships show increased risk of early death from all causes, risk for a heart attack and breast cancer. [178, 179,180]

Giving and receiving social support has been shown to lower blood pressure, inflammation and inflammatory markers in the blood. [181, 182]

A University of Washington study of college students discovered that the social dynamics of a group, such as whether one person dominates the group or works well with friends, affect academic performance. Students who reported a "dominator" in the group fared worse on the tests than those who didn't express that concern. Students who said they were comfortable in their group performed better than those who said they were less comfortable. The social support of the group can foster an atmosphere of confidence that spreads to all the members of the group. [183]

The Sicilian town is the original "social network". Families contribute to the lives and well-being of one another, hospitality never lacks along its streets, nor within its myriad of establishments. A friendly face is never hard to find and as a result, spirits are often high, regardless of circumstance. It may be that Sicilians long ago learned the secret many healthcare professionals have only recently realized: loneliness can be deadly.

Recent studies show that loneliness sparks a number of negative effects in the human body including hardening of the arteries, widespread inflammation (which is linked to onset of illness and disease), and even problems with learning and memory. Depression and loneliness are closely tied; studies of individuals suffering from depression show that the greater the sense of personal loneliness the more serious and debilitating is the depression.

We may be under the impression that devices and technology increase "connection" to one and other, but nothing could be farther from the truth according to research at the University of Chicago in 2015. All that time spent with Facebook, sending a tweet, clicking a YouTube video, or tapping a text is time spent alone. We are spending more time alone than ever before, and studies show a corresponding rate of increased loneliness with its clinical link to depression.

The quality of the marital relationship is a risk factor for heart disease, especially for men. The researchers found that women are not as negatively affected as men by a poor marital relationship, because women have larger social networks. [184]

Participating in group activities can significantly improve one's mental well-being. In Sicilian towns people frequently engage in group activities such as having coffee with family and friends, shopping in outdoor markets, and church activities. Researchers from East Anglia University, UK as part of the Sing Your Heart Out (SYHO) project, found that people who took part in a community singing group showed significantly improved mental health. [185]

Social support can help us meet our exercise goals. Having a small group of people to walk, hike or jog with, helps staying on track with exercise objectives. [186]

Clinical research proves what the heart already knows: social relationships combat ill health. Essentially, our social network can help us live longer.

Part III
THE 30-DAY PLAN

Chapter 13

THE 30-DAY SICILIAN SECRET DIET PLAN

Better Health, Four Weeks at a Time

Principal ingredients in the Sicilian Diet

THE SICILIAN CUISINE IS BASED on 5 fundamental elements: pasta, fish, cheeses, vegetables and sweets. Meat is a secondary element. It was and is eaten only occasionally and in small amounts. Meat was used mostly during a celebration and in unusual dishes. Meats from cows were rarely used because the few bovines that pastured in Sicily, were utilized to help the farmers to work the land. The meat would be eaten only when the animal was old and was no longer helpful. Because of the age of the animal the meat was hard and difficult to chew. The remedy to tough meat was to grind it, season it with spices and soften it with bread crumbs (meatballs, "polpette") or to slice it thin and pound it and sometimes stuff it (falsomagro, involtini, cutlets). Pork meat was more often present in the Sicilian tables (salami and sausage "salsiccia"), as were meats from goats and sheep. These animals were also essential in the production of cheeses (pecorino) and fresh and salted ricotta cheese, which is a traditional Sicilian specialty.

The Sicilian mild Mediterranean climate favors the growth of spices and herbs. Sicilian herbs are profoundly aromatic with an intense smell and flavor.

Herbs such as laurel, bay leaf ("addauro" in Sicilian), are largely used to dress meats, fish and preserves. Laurel is also used to make liquors and natural medicinal. The leaves have an antiseptic and gastrointestinal stimulant property. Cineole, a major compound in bay leaf can fight inflammation and aid wound healing. When used as tea, Laurel has a sedative effect and it is often prepared to treat stomach upset. The leaves have to be used only if dry because when green they can be slightly toxic.

Basil ("basilico" in Sicilian) is ubiquitous on the island and is used to infuse sauces and make pesto in its Genovese and Sicilian version. A winning combination is of basil with tomato (Pomodoro) sauce. Basil is rich in vitamin K, Manganese, Iron, Vitamin A and C. It contains calcium, magnesium and omega-3 fatty acids. Basil essential oils are used to treat cuts, wounds and skin infections. A plant of basil by the window will keep mosquitoes at bay.

The name oregano ("Riganu" in Sicilian), comes from two Greek words "oros" mountain and "ganos" splendor: the mountain splendor. It grows spontaneously around the mountain creating beautiful and aromatic green spots. It stimulates appetite and is used to marinate meats and fish and in salads and sauces. It is rich in antioxidants and has antibacterial and antiviral properties. It may help to lower cholesterol and improve gut health.

It is better to use small quantities of oregano in all food preparations because it will release a slightly bitter aroma.

Parsley, "Putrusino" in Sicilian, is possibly the herb that is mostly used all over the world. The Greeks and Romans used it abundantly in their cuisine and it continues to be greatly used today. It is rich in flavonoids, vitamin C, vitamin A, iron, manganese, calcium, phosphorus. It is a good herbal treatment for urinary tract infections and gout. It promotes a healthy heart and can help control arthritis.

Mint (mentuzza in Sicilian) grows wild all over the Sicilian countryside, rich in essential oils, flavonoids, tocopherols, carotenoids, choline and tannin. Great to cure indigestion and colds. It helps with nausea and headaches and promotes oral health.

It is widely used to enhance condiments, sauces, and liquors.

The capers or "ciappiru" in Sicilian, is the unopened flower of the caper bush that easily grows in every opening of a rock. It is usually preserved in salt or vinegar and used in many preparations, especially fish dishes. It is considered a good aphrodisiac and it is loaded with antioxidants. It can help with maintaining strong bones because capers are rich in vitamin K, calcium and magnesium. Capers can protect from allergies.

Capers harvested in Pantelleria, a small island off the coast of Sicily, have obtained the I.G.P rating (Indicazione Geografica Protetta) which is standard of high quality.

Garlic, "Agghiu" in Sicilian, has been known to humans since Egyptian times, it was loved by the Romans and hated by the Greeks. Garlic was used to treat many illnesses including urinary tract infections and yeast infections. Modern science confirms that garlic has the power to be antiseptic and can reduce cholesterol and blood pressure. It is helpful in removing heavy metals from the body.

It was used in large doses to cure children from intestinal worms and to cure conjunctivitis. Garlic is harvested in September and October and when kept in dry and well aerated storage can be used for the entire year.

Garlic enhances the flavor of most foods, it grows easily and has few pests that can attack it so that it is rarely sprayed with pesticides.

Garlic triumphs in many of the Sicilian dishes, whole, minced, pressed and roasted. It is utilized in vegetables, fish, meat and pasta dishes. Garlic is a powerful herbal medicine due mostly to one of its components, Alicen that can block the growth of several bacteria. Garlic is an effective antibiotic, antiviral and antifungal agent and is also a good antiseptic. Sicilian farmers used to carry garlic in their pockets in case of outbreaks of bacterial or viral infections. Garlic and onions work as blood thinners, preventing platelets aggregation, and are therefore helpful in heart disease. Raw garlic, mint and oregano will stimulate appetite.

Onion, "cipudda" in Sicilian, is one of the oldest vegetables we know. It is grown all over the world and was the basic staple for the nutrition of the Egyptian slaves. It is a powerful antioxidant rich in flavonoid compounds and quercetin and it has medicinal properties such as a diuretic, anti-bacterial, anti-viral, reduces inflammation and is a good vasodilator.

It is used for appetizers, entrées, side dishes, sauces, meat and fish dishes. In Sicily onions are often eaten raw with fresh bread, anchovies or pecorino cheese. The onion has the highest concentration of flavonoids in the outer layers, try not to over peel the onion.

Extra virgin olive oil contains essential vitamins and heart healthy monounsaturated fatty acids. It is rich in anti-oxidants, prevents gallstones and soothes gastric ulcers.

EVOO is rich in monounsaturated fats (oleic acid) and linoleic acid in proportions similar to human breast milk.

Cardiac mortality is lower in countries that use olive oil as the prevalent source of fat (Crete, Greece, Italy), probably because olive oil increases the good cholesterol (HDL) and reduces the bad (LDL) and has a beneficial blood thinning effect. Olive oil protects against osteoporosis, and has anti-cancer properties.

Sicilian cooks use Extra Virgin Olive Oil (EVOO) in many dishes, and they use it either raw or cooked. They have resisted the introduction of any other vegetable oil or butter in their diet.

Legumes - the meat of the peasants

The Sicilian climate and the nature of the soil are responsible for the abundant use of legumes in the Sicilian diet. They have been consumed by humans for over 10.000 years and they probably will be one the most respected foods of the future because they can substitute both cereals and meat due to their high protein content. Legumes contain large amounts of fiber, helpful for feeding the beneficial microorganisms in our guts, they decrease the speed that sugars enter our bloodstream (Glycemic Load) and help to increase bowel transit time resulting in decreased risk of constipation and hemorrhoids. A study done at Kentucky University, by Anderson, found that diabetes type II patients that were given a diet of whole grain bread and legumes reduced their insulin requirement by 38%. Legumes are rich in lecithin that facilitates the elimination of cholesterol via feces and reduces triglycerides. Legumes have a high and very bio absorbable protein content. They can be consumed regularly, and are a fundamental part of The Sicilian Secret Diet.

Fruits and vegetables

Humans have discovered fruit as the first and most important food. (Adam and Eve) It is the most vitalizing food because it is rich in simple carbohydrates, naturally purified water, fiber, minerals, vitamins, phytonutrients, and polyphenols. There are some nutritionists who believe that if we eat the sufficient amount of daily fruits and vegetables we do not need to drink additional water, because we can get all of the fluid we need from these foods. Seasonal fruits are the best because fruits are most nutritious when they are in season and our bodies have a seasonal capacity to absorb the fruits better when they are appropriately harvested. Fruits have powerful antioxidant properties that help us to prevent cancer and reduce cholesterol and triglycerides.

Fruits have high concentration of a phytonutrient called anthocyanins which have significant antioxidant function, they are anti-inflammatory, and help reduce the risk of heart disease and cancer.

Vegetables are a fundamental part of The Sicilian Secret Diet. Cultures around the world, whose diet emphasizes fruits, vegetables, whole grains and legumes have reduced rates of heart disease and cancers and have improved longevity when compared to cultures that do not adhere to this nutritional lifestyle. Vegetables contain high concentrations of chlorophyll which has powerful antioxidant and cancer fighting properties. The Sicilian Secret Diet emphasizes the consumption of a wide variety of colors of vegetables and fruits, because each color represents a different beneficial class of nutrients. In fact, vegetables contain thousands of beneficial phytonutrients which work alone and synergistically with each other to improve our health. It is the communion of all the beneficial substances present in fruits, vegetables, whole grains, herbs and legumes that promote health and not any one individual molecule. This is what the Sicilian diet does best, it unifies all the best nutrients in the most delicious dishes.

Vegetables contain among many other beneficial nutrients, glycosylates which are converted in the body to chemicals that can help the liver remove cancer-promoting toxins - this is one of the reasons that The Sicilian Secret Diet is naturally and continuously detoxifying.

Of all the vegetables and fruits that grow in the Sicilian land tomatoes are the most loved by Sicilians. Every family has its own tomato sauce that has been passed on through many generations. At the end of the summer my family, like most other families around us, would start the process of making tomato sauces and preserving them in jars for the winter, of drying tomatoes to make sun dried tomatoes and making tomato paste. I remember large tables of sliced tomatoes exposed to the sun during the day and brought back inside for the night. The smell was pungent and intense, it smelled of health and excitement. We were preparing a healthy treasure for our winter months when tomatoes would be no longer available.

Tomatoes contain Lycopene, a powerful antioxidant good for bone health.

Removing lycopene from post-menopausal women for just 4 weeks increases oxidative stress in the bones. Tomato varieties that offer the highest amount of antioxidants are: New Girl, Jet Star, Fantastic and First Lady.

Tomatoes promote heart health. They lower total cholesterol, bad cholesterol (LDL) and triglycerides. Tomato extract, often used in the Sicilian Diet, is a very good natural blood thinner helpful in preventing heart disease.

Whole grains - a vital food

Whole Grains have also been consumed by humans for over 10000 years. A serving of whole grains can provide energy for muscular activity for several hours and is a necessary part of a balanced diet. For thousands of years humans ate whole grains, however, in 1880 the first grain mill was invented and humans started consuming refined grains. White refined flour was regarded as food for the rich and was highly sought after. However, we know now that populations that use whole grains have significantly less diseases, and this "advance" of refined flour actually contains less nutritional value compared to whole grains because of the removal of the most nutritious part of the grain in the refining process. The germ and bran portion of the whole grain contains the best parts - the extremely rich concentration of phytonutrients such as elegiac acid and ferulic acid, which have been shown to prevent heart disease and other degenerative diseases such as dementia and cancers. Whole grains are also rich in fiber, polyphenols, vitamins, minerals, and protein. Regular consumption of whole grains helps to control obesity.

Pasta is the queen at Sicilian dinner tables, it is our gastronomic flag, always dressed up with the most fantastic sauce preparations. Pasta was handmade in Sicily much before Marco Polo returned from China. Grain was cultivated in Sicily in abundance and religious rituals have always accompanied the sowing and harvesting of these grains - it was considered a sacred food.

Durum flour, water, salt and a long energetic kneading of the dough creates a food that is simple, healthy and nutritious.

A good pasta dish brings a smile to everyone's face.

Durum flour is high in fiber, vitamin B, thiamine and folate, iron and magnesium, minerals that support heart health and blood sugar control. 100 gr of durum flour contains 13 gr of protein and less than 2 gr of fat.

Pasta is created in many shapes to accommodate different sauces. Short pasta adapts itself to most sauces while the long pastas are more adaptable for richer condiments such as carbonara amatriciana or vegetable sauces.

The thinner pastas such as vermicelli are best combined with light sauces such as fish sauces.

Bread is appreciated as an important food item because it provides nutrition and it is a food that helps achieve satiety. Sicilians never sit at the dinner table without bread. Bread has almost a religious veneration manifested by the simple gesture of kissing the piece of bread that accidentally falls on the floor and by preserving the crumbs to feed the animals or to make home-made bread crumbs instead of wasting them by throwing them away. Every Sicilian city bakes at least 10 different types of bread several times a day. Most Sicilians purchase freshly baked bread twice daily. As a child, it was mine and my cousin's job to walk down to the piazza, to find our chosen panificio (bread store) to buy the hot bread, just out of the oven, to bring home for our meal. While Hansel and Gretel disseminated their bread crumbs on the ground, we cover our steps picking at the hot bread... Few things will ever taste as good as that indulgence!

Starting your lifestyle change journey

I want to welcome you to my home in Sicily, a home from which I have never separated from in spite of my departure to North America at age twenty-four. As a proud and maybe stubborn Sicilian, I have kept the island culinary traditions alive, respecting flavors, obeying the law of seasonal recipes, shopping at the local farmer's markets, nurturing my own herbs and the few vegetables that I have been able to grow in my New Jersey backyard.

If you are reading this book today it is probably because you have already tried several diets and are looking for the new best one. This is not a diet book but a guide to a healthier lifestyle that does not involve calorie counts and it is an invitation to learn about nutrition through the wise guidance of our Sicilian ancestors.

Most of us get enthusiastic to start a diet and shortly after find ourselves becoming resentful or bored by the lack of flavor and excitement that most diets offer. Some of us accept having to start a diet the same way we would accept having to start a prison sentence. Flavor is a fundamental requisite for a successful diet. Sicilians believe that there are three fundamental rules for a good dish. It has to be "insucatu, oluruso and sapuritu", rich in condiment, smelling appetizing and full of flavor.

Learning to control portions is more helpful than counting calories. In this book we offer foods that are full of nutrition and flavor, that our ancestors have eaten for centuries and preserved for us. This is a journey in the present and in the past at the same time, it is a true lifestyle change that we can pass to future generations as our ancestors have done for us.

We will reinforce throughout the book tips that come in handy for succeeding at maintaining weight loss without feeling deprived, such as serving meals on small plates which allows for the brain to recognize abundance of food in a small but full dish.

This book is an attempt to help you to discover that engaging in a lifestyle change can be enjoyable. Success is making small changes and being able to sustain them over time.

A good diet is a fundamental part of a healthy lifestyle. Invite the whole family to embrace it, to participate in it and enjoy the process. We are not going to give you a new and undiscovered knowledge but we are going to share with you the wisdom collected through centuries by a population that has learned how to save and protect recipes that are simple, rich in flavor and that have great nutritional value.

Everybody's DNA holds a piece of Sicily, an island that has been conquered and occupied by many different cultures that have left behind culinary treasures that the Sicilians have saved and protected for all of us. This is a journey to discover some of that genetic past we are all connected with and the food that has helped us to become who we are.

There is a reason why Sicily is home to many centenarians.

Be encouraged to know that in spite of the common belief that 95% of diets fail, research has shown that 20% of overweight people can successfully sustain long-term weight loss. A successful weight loss is defined by the loss of at least 10% of initial body weight and having maintained the loss for at least 1 year. Even 5% loss of initial body weight is linked to improved health including reduction in cardiovascular risk factors such as diabetes, coronary disease, hypertension and high cholesterol.

Several factors can predict future weight gain.

A weight loss greater than 30% of initial body weight in one year places you at risk for future weight gain. Losing weight slowly helps to sustain weight loss. Observe your mood and your level of stress. Depressed people tend to regain weight more often than individuals who are not depressed. Greater levels of binge eating at the time of starting a diet also predicts weight gain. If depression and significant binge eating behaviors are present we recommend having the support of a mental health professional while starting your lifestyle change journey. Maintaining behavioral changes provides the greater ability to sustain weight loss over time.

You can succeed too

Ask yourself why you are considering entering this lifestyle change journey. Finding a good motivating factor helps to stay the course. Be mindful of the stress you are currently experiencing. Stress affects food choices and decrease the motivation to exercise. With stress, 65% of us eat more chocolate and candies; 56% eat more ice cream; 49% eat more cookies and only 8% of us eat more vegetables.

Starting a diet requires to be ready to let go of the foods that our brain recognizes as exciting and rewarding. Nutritious food is not a reward but a human need and right. Get started and try to stay the course for at least three to six weeks which is the amount of time that our brain requires for a new neural pathway to be established. Eventually the brain will be able to embrace this new lifestyle, recognize its value and naturally let go of wanting the processed foods that we have become accustomed to crave.

Join us and enter this process being aware that any change requires time, small changes are always a good start and are necessary to build on further changes. "All or nothing" approach to lifestyle change does not work for most people, start by taking small steps. Challenge your beliefs about dieting and start with setting up realistic and attainable goals.

What to buy at the supermarket can be the first challenge. It starts with paying attention to the food that we are used to buying, with observing how we feel when we let go of it and with being mindful of the changes that we are willing to make. Recognize the isles to avoid and become familiar with the isles that offer the foods that have the highest nutritional value.

Challenge your beliefs

1) "I cannot throw it away - I won't buy it anymore after I finish this box".

Open your cupboard. Look carefully at how many boxes of processed food it holds. Start reading the ingredients and understand the nutritional value they hold and lack. How many "snacks" are there? How many snacks do you and your family need?

Ask yourself what you are willing to throw away. Start removing the foods that have the least nutritional value and the highest content of saturated fats or sugar.

Observe how you feel, how hard or easy it is to let go. Observe without judging the experience and learn from the knowledge of your discovery. Food addiction is real. Understand your struggle, write it down, share it with someone you trust. Observe if you are making excuses of why you cannot throw things away, "I just bought it - I will finish this and then not buy it anymore- my kids have the right to have their snacks." Children have the same right to healthy and nutritious food that you have, they do not need processed snacks.

2) "I need to have my soda - I don't smoke, I don't drink, this is my only vice".

Open your refrigerator. Look carefully at how many sodas or juices it holds. Sodas, both regular and diet, have no nutritional value and are associated with increased risk of diabetes. Juices are processed foods. Artificial sweeteners can be harmful and also have no nutritional value. Diet sodas do not help people lose weight.

It takes just a few minutes to squeeze an orange or a lemon, to juice a pear or an apple and create our own unprocessed juice.

Fresh squeezed citrus and fruits retain all their nutritional value.

How many left over take-out food boxes, how much processed meats or processed cheese does your refrigerator contain? Do you have more than two varieties of fruits and vegetables?

Ask yourself what you can throw away and observe how you feel. What are the items that are harder to separate from?

3) "I do not like vegetables. My children will never eat vegetables".

Taste needs to be acquired. Start eating more of the vegetables you and your family already eat then introduce new ones. Our recipes are simple and will provide taste and flavor. Remember every time you eat it is an opportunity to feed the cells of your body the quality energy they require. Every time you eat empty calories it is a lost opportunity.

Every time you feel ready to let go of something (soda, potato chips, cookies, etc.) think about a healthy substitute. Substituting instead of just giving up something we have been accustomed to eat and enjoy is easier to accomplish than simply giving up something we love. For example, can you substitute soda with a fermented tea like kombucha, or flavor your water with natural fruit juice? Can you make a fruit salad and add honey and toasted nuts to substitute for desert?

4) "I don't have time to go shopping - I hate going to the supermarket".

Learn about farmers' markets near you, become familiar with the local produce and its nutritional value. Remember the power of good nutrition. A healthy meal provides you with energy, reduces anxiety and depression, improves the quality of sleep, improves your gut bacteria and it will help to reduce the amounts of any medicine you take.

People that shop at their farmer's market are healthier and thinner than people that solely shop at supermarkets. This also helps local small farms survive, which is a benefit to your community.

5) "I do not have time to cook".

Everyone can make time to cook.

What are the things that you engage in during the day that you can let go of to make time for cooking? Observe how much idle time you spend on the computer, how much time you spend watching TV and see if you can carve 20 minutes away from your favorite activity and dedicate that time to cooking. Can you engage your family members in cutting, chopping and cooking together? Remind yourself of the power of good nutrition.

6) "I do not have time to exercise".

Exercise does not have to be intense or strenuous in order to work. If a sedentary person starts with exercising 15 minutes / day, he or she can decrease the risk of death by 14% and increase life expectancy by three years.

The body will slow its metabolism when we crash diet and with aging, our metabolism will also slow down partly due to the loss of lean muscle mass. The more we crash diet the more we slow down our metabolism. Paradoxically, eating a good balanced and nutritionally rich diet is a good way to lose weight without lowering your metabolism. Also, exercise will increase metabolism facilitating weight loss.

Go through your day and observe how you have used your time. Did you have 15 minutes to take a walk? Taking a 15-minute walk or dancing to your favorite song is a good way to start exercising. Observe what is the time of the day that you have most energy. Are you a morning person or a night person? Finding the motivation to exercise comes easier if you engage in the activity with a friend or a dog.

7) Be mindful.

Attentive eating reduces calorie intake without the need for conscious calorie counting.

Avoid distractions while eating such as watching TV or looking at your phone or computer. Increase awareness of the food you are consuming. For example, the simple recall of the food eaten during your last meal can help reduce the calorie intake during the next meal.

We are able to make small changes and we are able to maintain them.

Let your motivation remind you of your goals. We deserve to be healthy and to feel strong.

- **We can sit down at the dinner table for every meal instead of eating in the car or eating in front of a screen. Can this be a small attainable goal for you to set for today?**

- **We can eat slowly and savor our food. If we chew every bite 20 to 40 times we will end up eating 1/4 to 1/2 of what we normally eat and since digestion begins in the mouth the food will be better absorbed and cause less gastrointestinal disturbances. Eating slowly gets in the way of eating too much.**

- **We can wait 20 minutes before taking a second serving. It takes 20 minutes for our stomach to communicate to our brain that it is full and during those 20 minutes we can eat more calories than our body needs. This may be one of the reasons that there is less heart disease and other ailments in Sicily, because Sicilians tend to eat the largest meal of the day at midday and they eat it slowly with friends and family.**

Chapter 14

THE 30-DAY SICILIAN SECRET DIET PLAN

BEFORE GETTING STARTED, READ THIS short list of simple suggestions that might help you embrace the changes that you will implement. These changes can help you to sustain a lifestyle that will improve your physical and mental health and add a few healthy years to your life.

This nutritional change does not require you to count calories or points, it is a diet that trusts the power of good and tasty food. It requires you to be mindful of portion sizes and have patience with shopping and preparing food.

I tried to choose the quickest and simplest recipes that should not require more than 20/30 minutes to prepare.

Goals:

1. **Eat 3 to 5 meals per day, always in small portions and serve all the food in small plates.**
2. **Place everything you will eat for that meal in one dish without picking during the meal.**
3. **Eat sitting down at the dinner table, set placemat, avoid watching TV or the use of electronics.**

4. Eat slowly and pay attention to what you eat. Wait 20 minutes before taking a second serving.

5. Eat the food offered to you by the seasons and shop in local farmer markets.

6. Buy frozen vegetables and frozen fruits off season.

7. Eat in colors. Every color represents a different vitamin and different mineral and nutritional supplement.

8. Eat variety of foods. A diet that offers variety is easier to maintain and is more healthful. Food has to be appealing to the eyes as much as to the palate.

9. Eat whole grains, legumes, nuts, seeds, fruits and vegetables every day.

10. Legumes, oats, barley, garlic, onions, grapes, orange peel and anise, are some of the foods that help control the production of cholesterol in the liver.

11. Eat quality red meat less than once per week.

12. Eat fish two to three times per week, always look for wild, small and cold water ocean fish.

13. Eat quality chicken no more than 2 times per week.

14. Eat 1 egg 2 to 3 times per week.

15. Drink one glass of water or one cup of organic tea 20 minutes before every meal.

16. Drink one to three cups of coffee or green or black tea per day, (if you enjoy it) never later than 2 pm.

17. Drink only organic tea. Use honey and not sugar for your tea. Use 1 TBSP of whole milk or almond milk, and no more than 1 tsp of unrefined cane sugar for your coffee.

18. Drink one small glass of wine with your dinner if you enjoy it.

19. Drink herbal tea with raw honey and lemon before bedtime - chamomile tea is great choice at bedtime

20. Be active and engage in any physical activity that is enjoyable to you, activity does not have to be strenuous but let your body move every day, it will be forever grateful to you.

21. Sleep 7 to 9 hours every night.

22. Try to eat most of your calories at the beginning of the day, you can include your snack with your meal, or you can skip your snack.

23. Allow for at least 12 to 14 hours of fasting time which means that if you eat your last meal/snack at 7 pm you should not have breakfast before 7 or 9 am. The body starts burning fat only after 10 hours of fasting.

24. Expose yourself with your eyes open to the early morning light (7 am-11 am) for 5-10 minutes. This will reset your circadian rhythm, increase your natural melatonin and help you sleep better at night. You can combine this with meditation (Headspace App) or breathing exercises (Pranayama Universal Breathing app).

Portion sizes

- All pasta portions are 100 gr (3.5 ounces) uncooked per person

- All rice portions are ½ a cup uncooked, 1 cup cooked per person

- All meat portions are 100 gr (3.5 ounces) uncooked per person

- All fish portions are 220 gr (8 ounces) uncooked per person

- All legumes and grains portions are 50 gr (1.8 ounces) uncooked per person, 1 cup cooked

- Make legumes and grains on the weekend. They can be stored in the refrigerator up to 5 days or frozen in portion sizes in Ziploc bags for up to 3 months. When you are ready to eat them place in a pot with ¼ water and reheat.**Grill your vegetables on the weekend.** They can be stored in the refrigerator for 5 days or frozen for one month.

Shopping list

Always in the pantry:

- Good quality extra virgin olive oil; aged vinegar; black and green olives; capers; San Marzano tomatoes cans, dry beans, lentils, chickpeas, fava beans, onions white and red, garlic, oregano, rosemary, basil, parsley, bay leaves; raw honey; unrefined cane sugariness; ancient grain pasta; wild rice; walnuts; almonds; cashew; flax seeds; chia seeds; bulgur wheat; farro (spelt); quinoa; kamut; potatoes; sweet potatoes. Dark chocolate, at least 70% cocoa and 30% organic sugar cane.

Always in the refrigerator and freezer

- Tomatoes
- Mixed greens, sprouts
- Seasonal vegetables to cook every day such as: broccoli, cauliflower, string beans, spinach, collard greens, chicory, artichokes, peas, peppers, eggplant, leeks
- Seasonal fruit

- Yogurt, organic pasteurized (avoid ultra-pasteurized milk or yogurt) grass fed whole milk or almond milk, aged cheese such as pecorino or Parmesan cheese, free range organic eggs.
- Protein of choice
- Add chia seeds and flax seeds and sprouts to your salads and granola daily

What to look for when shopping:

Always organic

- Strawberries, Spinach, Nectarines, Apples, Peaches, Pears, Cherries, Grapes, Celery, Cherry tomatoes, Sweet bell peppers, Potato.

- These are the fruits and vegetable that contain the highest amount of pesticides and toxins including traces of DDT which is a neurotoxic insecticide banned in the USA.

- According to the 2017 Environmental working group study, a single strawberry sample contains 20 different pesticides.

2) Ok to buy not organic

- The food items that contain the least amount of pesticides are: Sweet corn, Avocados, Pineapples, Cabbage, Onion, Frozen Sweet Peas, Papayas, Asparagus, Mangoes, Eggplant, Honeydew, Kiwi, Cantaloupe, Cauliflower, Grapefruit.

3) Meats

- Choose grass fed and grass finished meats. Grass finished means that the animal has been fed grass for its entire life. Grass fed label does not guarantee that the animal has been grass fed for its entire life.

- Prefer lean cuts such as "round", "loin", "sirloin".

- Buy "choice", "select" grades of beef rather than "prime".

- Prefer lean veal, lamb, buffalo or wild game such as rabbit, pheasant, venison, wild duck.

- Bake, broil, stew or grill your meats.

- Choose poultry without skin.

4) Fish

- Choose fish high in omega 3 such as mackerel, lake trout, herring, sardines, albacore, salmon.

- Avoid shark, swordfish, tilefish (golden bass or golden snapper), and king mackerel which contain high levels of mercury.

5) Yogurt

- Choose plain yogurt free of sugar and sweeteners. If you do not like plain yogurt add your own fruit, jam, honey, maple sugar. In order for a yogurt to serve as a good probiotic it needs to contain at least 1,000,000 living bacteria per gram. The live bacteria in yogurt is labeled as CFU. A good yogurt should have a LAC seal (live and active cultures). The bacteria in the yogurt become metabolically active once we ingest them and support proper digestion and absorption of nutrients. Yogurt possibly converts food sugar into short chain fatty acids used as energy for the endothelial cells and prevents leaky gut. The content of lactose is much smaller in yogurt compared to milk because the live bacteria break down lactose.

- Yogurt has a protein to carbohydrate ratio that makes it an ideal snack that can promote weight loss by boosting metabolism and minimizing hunger pain

- Best yogurts: Wallaby organic Greek plain; Maple Hill Creamery Greek yogurt; Fage Total 2% Greek yogurt; Brown Cow; Stonyfield Organic Greek whole milk Plain yogurt; Organic Valley Grass milk yogurt; Siggi's yogurt.

6) Extra Virgin Olive Oil (EVOO)

- Choose olive oils that have the International Olive Oil Council (IOC) seal.

- All olive oils are not created equal. Best olive oils are the oils that are milled within 24 hrs. of the olives harvest and are extracted by mechanical means and not by heat or chemicals. The unfiltered version, which is cloudy, is preferred because it will contain more polyphenols and phytonutrients.

- This is a list of some of the olive oils that have failed to meet EVOO standards:

- Bertolli, Carapelli, Colavita, Star, Filippo Berio, Mazzola, Mazzetta, Newman's own, Safeway, Whole foods.

- This is the list of the olive oils that have passed the EVOO standards:

- Bariani olive oil, Corto olive oil, Cobram Estate, California olive Ranch, Kirkland Organic, Lucero (Ascolano), Whole foods California 365, Ellora extra virgin, Trader Joe's California Estate,

7) Vinegar

- Choose aged wine vinegar of great quality, you need only a small amount for dressing. Aged balsamic vinegar is very expensive but you need only a few drops for flavor.

- You can substitute vinegar with fresh squeezed organic lemon or apple cider vinegar.

8) Bread

- Choose bread that has whole grains and only flour, yeast, seeds, water and salt as ingredients.

- Bread can be sliced and frozen for up to one week to provide convenient access to daily portions.

- Unless you have Celiac Disease or true gluten intolerance (1% of population), gluten is good for you! It helps lower the risk of type 2 diabetes. A research published in the Journal of Diabetology followed gluten intake and diabetes incidence rates published in the Nurses' Health study and in the Health Professional Follow up Study. Women who ate foods rich in barley, wheat and rye, showed a reduced risk for diabetes type II compared to the women who did not.

- A meta-analysis study that included more than 400,000 participants, showed that a low carbohydrate diet (40% or less calories from carbs), had the same mortality risk than a high carbohydrate diet (70 % or more calories from carbs). A diet that offers 50/55% carbohydrates is associated with minimal mortality risk and greater life expectancy. (The Lancet Public health.)

Chapter 15
DAILY ROUTINES

Daily Routines of The 30-Day Sicilian Secret Diet

Day 1

Good morning!

Start your day thinking about **3** things you are grateful for.

Don't forget to smile, laugh, dance, walk, skip, jump and meditate today. Exercise for **30** minutes if you can. (Recipes start on page **215**.)

Breakfast :
- ⅓ cup Homemade Granola (see recipe) or store bought granola
- ½ cup whole processed milk (avoid ultra-processed milk)
- 1 cup seasonal fruit
- coffee or tea optional

Snack:

- 1 cup yogurt (always choose yogurts that have the highest amount of active culture and the wider variety of bacteria)
- coffee or tea optional

Lunch:

- 1 slice whole grain bread
- Roasted Peppers (see recipe)
- Marinated Grilled, Free-Range chicken (see recipe) (3.5 ounces)
- mixed green salad with one Tbsp of EVOO and 1 Tbsp of vinegar, salt, pepper

Snack:

- ¼ cup (toasted) nuts
- coffee or tea optional

Dinner:

- Farro Parmesan Risotto with Parmesan cheese (see recipe) (portion size 1 cup cooked farro)
- Cannellini Bean and Red Onion Salad (see recipe) (1 cup cooked beans)
- 1 glass wine optional

Snack: (no later than 7 pm)

- 1 cup of mixed berries and 1 tsp manuka honey

It is time to end your day and unwind.

Shut all electronics off 1-2 hours before bedtime.

Go through your day and think about 3 good things that have happened to you and be grateful.

Make sure that you sleep 7 to 9 hours tonight.

Find 10 minutes to stretch and meditate before going to bed.
Have a good night.

Day 2

Good morning! Start your day thinking about 3 things you are grateful for. Don't forget to dance, walk, skip, jump, meditate today.

Breakfast:
- 1 cup Oatmeal (see recipe) with golden raisins, citrus zest and 1 Tbsp maple syrup (1 cup cooked oatmeal)
- coffee or tea optional

Snack:
- 1 cup seasonal fruit

Lunch:
- Grilled Salmon (see recipe) with Salmoriglio sauce (see recipe) (serving size 8 ounces)
- Lentil and Barley Salad or Summer Tomatoes, Red Onion Salad (see recipe)

Snack:
- 1 cup yogurt
- coffee or tea optional

Dinner:
- Ancient Grain Pasta Salad (see recipe) (serving size 100 gr uncooked pasta)
- steamed broccoli with ½ Tbsp EVOO and fresh lemon juice, salt and pepper
- Roasted Eggplants and Zucchini (see recipe)
- 1 glass of wine optional

Snack:

- 1 cup baby carrots and 1 Tbsp hummus

It is time to end your day and unwind.

Shut all electronics off 1-2 hours before bedtime.

Go through your day and think about 3 good things that have happened to you and be grateful.

Make sure that you sleep 7 to 9 hours tonight.

Find 10 minutes to stretch and meditate before going to bed.
Have a good night.

Day 3

Good morning! Start your day thinking about 3 things you are grateful for. Don't forget to dance, walk, skip, jump, meditate today.

Breakfast:

- 1 cup yogurt
- 1 cup seasonal fruit,
- 1 Tbsp manuka honey
- coffee or tea optional

Snack:

- 1 hard-boiled egg with 1 tsp of Homemade Mayonnaise (see recipe)

Lunch:

- Kamut Chickpea Salad with Summer Tomatoes, Red Onion Salad (see recipe) (serving size 1 cup of cooked kamut)
- Sautéed Spinach in EVOO (see recipe), garlic sprinkled with 1 Tbsp pecorino cheese

Snack:

- 1 cup of celery, 1 cup of carrots, 1 Tbsp of Homemade Mayonnaise (see recipe) and 1 tsp of mustard
- coffee or tea optional

Dinner:
- ½ Baked Cornish Game Hen (see recipe)
- 1 small potato (can be substitute with sweet potato) baked or steamed
- with ½ Tbsp of butter and 1 Tbsp of Parmesan cheese
- mixed green salad
- 1 glass wine optional

Snack:
- roasted nuts toasted with a sprinkle of unrefined sugar

It is time to end your day and unwind.

Shut all electronics off 1-2 hours before bedtime.

Go through your day and think about 3 good things that have happened to you and be grateful.

Make sure that you sleep 7 to 9 hours tonight.

Find 10 minutes to stretch and meditate before going to bed.
Have a good night.

Day 4

Good morning! Start your day thinking about 3 things you are grateful for. Don't forget to dance, walk, skip, jump, meditate today.

Breakfast:

- Bulgur Wheat with Roasted Almonds (see recipe), brown sugar, cinnamon and berries (serving size ½ cup of cooked bulgur)
- coffee or tea optional

Snack:

- 1 cup yogurt

Lunch:

- Minestrone Soup (see recipe) (1 soup bowl)
- Grilled Vegetables (see recipe) sprinkled with Gorgonzola cheese
- 1 slice whole grain bread

Snack:

- 1 cup seasonal fruit
- coffee or tea optional

Dinner:
- Polenta (see recipe) (corn grits or stone ground coarse cornmeal) cooked in chicken or vegetable broth) and 1 Tbsp Parmesan cheese (serving size 1 cup of cooked polenta)
- Sautéed Mushrooms (see recipe)
- 1 glass wine optional

Snack:
- 1 Poached Pear in wine (see recipe)

It is time to end your day and unwind.

Shut all electronics off 1-2 hours before bedtime.

Go through your day and think about 3 good things that have happened to you and be grateful.

Make sure that you sleep 7 to 9 hours tonight.

Find 10 minutes to stretch and meditate before going to bed.
Have a good night.

Day 5

Good morning! Start your day thinking about 3 things to be grateful for. Don't forget to dance, walk, skip, jump, meditate today.

Breakfast:

- smoothie: ½ cup spinach, ½ cup broccoli, ½ cup kale, 1 tomato, 1 apple, ½ cup yogurt , 1 Tbsp of manuka honey, ½ Tbsp flax seeds, ½ Tbsp chia seeds. Place all ingredients into a blender.
- coffee or tea optional

Snack:

- 1 hard-boiled egg with 1 tsp Homemade Mayonnaise (see recipe) and mustard

Lunch:

- Grilled Shrimp (see recipe) with Salmoriglio sauce (see recipe) (3.5 ounces)
- mixed green salad with 1 Tbsp vinegar, 1 Tbsp EVOO, salt and pepper
- Cannellini Beans and Red Onion Salad (see recipe) (1 cup cooked beans)

Snack:

- 1 cup seasonal fruit
- coffee or tea optional

Dinner:

- Ancient Grain Pasta Salad with Pesto Sauce (see recipe) (serving size 1 cup uncooked pasta)
- Grilled Vegetables (see recipe) sprinkled with goat cheese
- 1 glass wine optional

Snack:

- 3 ounces dark chocolate (at least 70% cacao, 30% organic cane sugar)
- dark chocolate consumption reduces stress and inflammation, improves memory, immunity and mood!

It is time to end your day and unwind.

Shut all electronics off 1-2 hours before bedtime.

Go through your day and think about 3 good things that have happened to you and be grateful.

Make sure that you sleep 7 to 9 hours tonight.

Find 10 minutes to stretch and meditate before going to bed.
Have a good night.

Day 6

Good morning! Start your day thinking about 3 things you are grateful for. Don't forget to dance, walk, skip, jump, meditate today.

Breakfast:
- Grits (see recipe), Greek yogurt, manuka honey, orange peel (serving size 1 cup cooked Grits)
- coffee or tea optional

Snack:
- ¼ cup nuts

Lunch:
- Arugula, Avocado Salad (see recipe)
- Chickpea Soup (see recipe)
- 1 slice whole grain bread

Snack:
- 1 cup seasonal fruit
- coffee or tea optional

Dinner:
- Pan Seared Flounder (see recipe) (serving size 8 ounces)
- Peas and Artichoke Stew (see recipe) (serving size 1 cup)
- Summer Tomatoes, Red Onion Salad (see recipe)
- 1 glass of wine optional

Snack:

- ½ cup hot milk with 2 ounces dark chocolate

It is time to end your day and unwind.

Shut all electronics off 1-2 hours before bedtime.

Go through your day and think about 3 good things that have happened to you and be grateful.

Make sure that you sleep 7 to 9 hours tonight.

Find 10 minutes to stretch and meditate before going to bed.
Have a good night.

Day 7

Good morning! Start your day thinking about 3 things you are grateful for. Don't forget to dance, walk, skip, jump, meditate today.

Breakfast:
- Creamy Farro with Roasted Grapes (see recipe) (serving size 1 cup of cooked farro)
- coffee or tea optional

Snack:
- yogurt

Lunch:
- Ancient Grain Pasta Salad with Broccoli and Cauliflower Pasta Sauce (see recipe) [serving size 100 grams (3.5 ounces) of uncooked pasta]
- steamed broccoli di rapa with 1 Tbsp EVOO and minced garlic

Snack:
- 1 cup seasonal fruit
- coffee or tea optional

Dinner:
- Onion, Pecorino Frittata (see recipe)
- Bulgur Wheat, Lentil, Olive Salad (see recipe)
- 1 slice whole grain bread
- 1 glass wine optional

Snack:

- ¼ cup toasted nuts and 1 tsp manuka honey

It is time to end your day and unwind.

Shut all electronics off 1-2 hours before bedtime.

Go through your day and think about 3 good things that have happened to you and be grateful.

Make sure that you sleep 7 to 9 hours tonight.

Find 10 minutes to stretch and meditate before going to bed.
Have a good night.

CONGRATULATIONS!

YOU HAVE MADE THROUGH THE first week!

Please take a moment to congratulate yourself and observe without judging the steps that were easy to take and the ones you struggled with. Write it down, talk with someone you trust.

What can you do different and better this week. Are you ready for your second week?

Let's start together again.

Day 8

Good morning! Start your day thinking about 3 things you are grateful for. Don't forget to dance, walk, skip, jump, meditate today.

Breakfast:

- smoothie: 1 cup kale, ½ cucumber, 1 cup spinach, 1 green apple, 1 clove of garlic, 1 Tbsp olive oil, ½ cup yogurt, 1 Tbsp manuka honey, ½ Tbsp flax seeds. Place all ingredients into a blender.
- coffee or tea optional

Snack:

- 1 cup carrots, 1 cup celery with 1 Tbsp balsamic vinegar and ½ Tbsp EVOO, salt and pepper to taste

Lunch:

- Kamut Chickpea Salad or Lentil and Barley Salad (see recipes) (serving size 1 cup cooked)
- Sautéed Spinach (see recipe)
- 3 ounces pecorino cheese

Snack:

- 1 cup seasonal fruit
- coffee or tea optional

Dinner:
- Baked Chicken or Beef Cutlets (see recipe) (serving size 3.5 ounces)
- String Beans and Potato Salad (see recipe)
- 1 glass wine optional

Snack:
- ½ cup nuts toasted with a sprinkle of brown sugar

It is time to end your day and unwind.

Shut all electronics off 1-2 hours before bedtime.

Go through your day and think about 3 good things that have happened to you and be grateful.

Make sure that you sleep 7 to 9 hours tonight.

Find 10 minutes to stretch and meditate before going to bed.
Have a good night.

Day 9

Good morning! Start your day thinking about 3 things you are grateful for. Don't forget to dance, walk, skip, jump, meditate today.

Breakfast:

- 1 soft boiled egg
- 1 slice of whole grain bread with 1 tsp fresh jam
- ½ cup whole milk
- coffee or tea optional

Snack:

- 1 cup seasonal fruit

Lunch:

- Cannellini Bean and Red Onion Salad (see recipe)
- Steamed Cauliflower (see recipe) with 1 Tbsp EVOO and fresh lemon juice

Snack:

- ½ cup nuts
- coffee or tea optional

Dinner:

- Organic Free-Range Chicken Soup (see recipe) (serving size one soup bowl)
- 1 baked potato with 1 Tbsp olive oil, chopped fresh parsley and 1 clove of minced garlic
- mixed green salad with cherry tomatoes (1 Tbsp vinegar, 1 Tbsp EVOO, salt and pepper to taste)
- 1 glass wine optional

Snack:

- 3 ounces dark chocolate

It is time to end your day and unwind.

Shut all electronics off 1-2 hours before bedtime.

Go through your day and think about 3 good things that have happened to you and be grateful.

Make sure that you sleep 7 to 9 hours tonight.

Find 10 minutes to stretch and meditate before going to bed.
Have a good night.

Day 10

Good morning! Start your day thinking about **3** things you are grateful for. Don't forget to dance, walk, skip, jump, meditate today.

Breakfast:

- smoothie: 1 cup spinach, 1 carrot, 1 cup of mixed berries, 1 banana, ½ cup yogurt, 1 clove garlic, 1 tsp manuka honey, ½ Tbsp flax seeds, ½ Tbsp chia seeds. Place all ingredients into a blender.
- coffee or tea optional

Snack:

- ½ cup yogurt, ¼ cup nuts

Lunch:

- Fava Bean or Spinach Creamy Soup (see recipes) (serving size one soup bowl)
- 1 slice of whole grain bread
- steamed broccoli with 1 Tbsp EVOO and squeezed fresh lemon juice.

Snack:

- 1 cup seasonal fruit
- coffee or tea optional

Dinner:

- Marinated Grilled Pork Chop (see recipe) (serving size **3.5** ounces)
- mixed green salad
- Lentil and Barley Salad (see recipe) (serving size **1** cup cooked farro and lentils)
- **1** glass wine optional

Snack:

- ½ cup warm whole milk

It is time to end your day and unwind.

Shut all electronics off **1-2** hours before bedtime.

Go through your day and think about **3** good things that have happened to you and be grateful.

Make sure that you sleep **7** to **9** hours tonight.

Find **10** minutes to stretch and meditate before going to bed.
Have a good night.

Day 11

Good morning! Start your day thinking about 3 things you are grateful for. Don't forget to dance, walk, skip, jump, meditate today.

Breakfast:

- Spinach Frittata (see recipe)
- 1 slice whole grain bread
- 1 fresh squeezed orange juice
- coffee or tea optional

Snack:

- 1 yogurt

Lunch:

- Minestrone Soup (see recipe)
- Roasted Eggplant and Zucchini (see recipe)

Snack:

- ¼ cup nuts
- coffee or tea optional

Dinner:

- Baked Wild Salmon with Mustard (see recipe) (serving size 8 ounces)
- Bean and Quinoa Salad (see recipe) (serving size 1 cup cooked quinoa)
- mixed green salad with 1 Tbsp vinegar, 1 Tbsp EVOO, salt and pepper to taste
- 1 glass of wine optional

Snack:

- 1 grilled apple with 1 tsp honey and ½ Tbsp pistachio

It is time to end your day and unwind.

Shut all electronics off 1-2 hours before bedtime.

Go through your day and think about 3 good things that have happened to you and be grateful.

Make sure that you sleep 7 to 9 hours tonight.

Find 10 minutes to stretch and meditate before going to bed.
Have a good night.

Day 12

Good morning! Start your day thinking about 3 things you are grateful for. Don't forget to dance, walk, skip, jump, meditate today.

Breakfast:

- Oatmeal (see recipe), ½ cup raisins, ½ apple, ¼ cup walnuts, 1 Tbsp maple syrup (serving size 1 cup of cooked oatmeal)
- coffee or tea optional

Snack:

- 1 cup yogurt

Lunch:

- Ancient Grain Pasta Salad with Classic Tomato Sauce (see recipes) and pecorino cheese [serving size 100 grams (3.5 ounces) of uncooked pasta]
- mixed green salad with 1 Tbsp of vinegar, 1 Tbsp EVOO, salt and pepper to taste
- Orange Fennel Sicilian Salad (see recipe)

Snack:

- ¼ cup nuts
- coffee or tea optional

Dinner:

- Mixed Bean Soup (see recipe) (serving size 1 soup bowl)
- 1 slice whole grain bread
- Sautéed Spinach (see recipe)
- 1 glass wine optional

Snack:

- 2 ounces dark chocolate

It is time to end your day and unwind.

Shut all electronics off 1-2 hours before bedtime.

Go through your day and think about 3 good things that have happened to you and be grateful.

Make sure that you sleep 7 to 9 hours tonight.

Find 10 minutes to stretch and meditate before going to bed.
Have a good night.

Day 13

Good morning! Start your day thinking about 3 things you are grateful for. Don't forget to dance, walk, skip, jump, meditate today.

Breakfast:

- Bulgur Wheat with Roasted Almonds (see recipe) with toasted nuts, maple syrup and berries (serving size 1 cup uncooked bulgur)
- coffee or tea optional

Snack:

- 1 cup yogurt

Lunch:

- String Bean, Potato and Egg Salad (see recipe)
- Grilled Vegetables (see recipe)
- 1 slice whole grain bread

Snack:

- raw vegetables (carrots, celery, radicchio) and 2 Tbsp Eggplant Spread (see recipe)
- coffee or tea optional

Dinner:

- Grouper with Capers and Kalamata Olives (see recipe) (serving size 8 ounces)
- mixed green salad with 1 Tbsp vinegar, 1 Tbsp EVOO, salt and pepper to taste
- Wild Rice and Parmigiano Cheese, (see recipe) (serving size 1 cup cooked rice)
- 1 glass wine optional

Snack:

- 1 Poached Pear

It is time to end your day and unwind.

Shut all electronics off 1-2 hours before bedtime.

Go through your day and think about 3 good things that have happened to you and be grateful.

Make sure that you sleep 7 to 9 hours tonight.

Find 10 minutes to stretch and meditate before going to bed.
Have a good night.

Day 14

Good morning! Start your day thinking about 3 things you are grateful for. Don't forget to dance, walk, skip, jump, meditate today.

Breakfast:

- 1 cup cooked Oatmeal (see recipe), cup dates, ½ cup berries, 1 tsp honey or 1 tsp maple syrup
- coffee or tea optional

Snack:

- 1 cup seasonal fruit

Lunch:

- Ancient Grain Pasta Salad with Pesto Sauce (see recipe) [serving size 100 grams (3.5 ounces) uncooked pasta and 2 Tbsp Pesto Sauce (see recipe)]
- mixed green salad with 1 Tbsp vinegar, 1 Tbsp EVOO, salt and pepper to taste

Snack:

- cup nuts
- coffee or tea optional

Dinner:

- Fava Bean, Chicoria or Spinach Creamy Soup (see recipes) (serving size 1 bowl of soup)
- 1 slice whole grain bread
- 3 ounces pecorino or Parmesan cheese

Snack:

- 1 cup yogurt

It is time to end your day and unwind.

Shut all electronics off 1-2 hours before bedtime.

Go through your day and think about 3 good things that have happened to you and be grateful.

Make sure that you sleep 7 to 9 hours tonight.

Find 10 minutes to stretch and meditate before going to bed.
Have a good night.

CONGRATULATIONS!

YOU HAVE MADE TO THE first two weeks! Can you feel the changes in your body, do you have more energy, are you sleeping better, are you feeling stronger? Take a few minutes to acknowledge challenges and success. Think about the challenges and consider a reasonable plan that might help you to overcome them. Think about the success, feel proud.

Day 15

Good morning! Start your day thinking about 3 things you are grateful for. Don't forget to dance, walk, skip, jump, meditate today.

Breakfast:

- Spinach Frittata (see recipe)
- 1 slice whole grain bread with 1 tsp jam or 1 tsp honey
- cappuccino (½ cup milk)

Snack:

- 2 cups raw vegetables with 2 Tbsp hummus

Lunch:

- Ancient Grain Pasta Salad (see recipe) [serving size 100 grams (3.5 ounces) uncooked pasta]
- Marinated Grilled, Free-Range Chicken (3.5 ounces)
- mixed green salad with 1 Tbsp vinegar, 1 Tbsp EVOO, salt and pepper to taste

Snack:

- 1 cup yogurt
- coffee or tea optional

Dinner:

- Minestrone Soup (see recipe) (serving size 1 soup bowl)
- Grilled Vegetables (see recipe)
- 1 slice whole grain bread
- 1 glass wine optional

Snack:

- 2 ounces dark chocolate

It is time to end your day and unwind.

Shut all electronics off 1-2 hours before bedtime.

Go through your day and think about 3 good things that have happened to you and be grateful.

Make sure that you sleep 7 to 9 hours tonight.

Find 10 minutes to stretch and meditate before going to bed.
Have a good night.

Day 16

Good morning! Start your day thinking about 3 things you are grateful for. Don't forget to dance, walk, skip, jump, meditate today.

Breakfast:

- 1 cup yogurt with 2 Tbsp Homemade Granola (see recipe) and 1 tsp honey
- 1 cup seasonal fruit
- coffee or tea optional

Snack:

- 1 cup raw vegetables with 2 Tbsp Eggplant Spread (see recipe)

Lunch:

- Ancient Grain Pasta Salad (see recipe) with broccoli anchovy and raisins [serving size 100 grams (3.5 ounces) uncooked pasta]
- mixed green salad with 1 Tbsp vinegar, 1 Tbsp EVOO, salt and pepper to taste

Snack:

- 1 cup seasonal fruit
- coffee or tea optional

Dinner:

- Branzino (see recipe) with Salmoriglio sauce (see recipe) (serving size 8 ounces)
- Cannellini Bean and Red Onion Salad (see recipe) (serving size 1 cup cooked)
- 1 slice ancient grain or whole grain bread
- 1 glass wine optional

Snack:

- ¼ cup toasted nuts sprinkled with raw cane sugar

It is time to end your day and unwind.

Shut all electronics off 1-2 hours before bedtime.

Go through your day and think about 3 good things that have happened to you and be grateful.

Make sure that you sleep 7 to 9 hours tonight.

Find 10 minutes to stretch and meditate before going to bed.
Have a good night.

Day 17

Good morning! Start your day thinking about 3 things you are grateful for. Don't forget to dance, walk, skip, jump, meditate today.

Breakfast:

- 1 slice of whole grain bread with 1 tsp jam
- cappuccino with 1 cup of whole milk
- fresh squeezed orange juice

Snack:

- ¼ cup nuts

Lunch:

- Cannellini Bean and Red Onion Salad (see recipe) (serving size 1 cup cooked)
- Marinated Grilled Sirloin (serving size 3 ounces)
- mixed green salad with 1 Tbsp vinegar, 1 Tbsp EVOO, salt and pepper to taste

Snack:

- 1 cup seasonal fruit
- coffee or tea optional

Dinner:

- Lentil Soup (see recipe) (serving size 1 soup bowl)
- Steamed Cauliflower with 1 Tbsp EVOO and fresh squeezed lemon juice, salt and pepper to taste
- 1 glass wine optional

Snack:

- 2 ounces dark chocolate

It is time to end your day and unwind.

Shut all electronics off 1-2 hours before bedtime.

Go through your day and think about 3 good things that have happened to you and be grateful.

Make sure that you sleep 7 to 9 hours tonight.

Find 10 minutes to stretch and meditate before going to bed.
Have a good night.

Day 18

Good morning! Start your day thinking about 3 things you are grateful for. Don't forget to dance, walk, skip, jump, meditate today.

Breakfast:

- 1 slice whole grain bread and 1 tsp jam
- 1 cup seasonal fruit
- coffee or tea optional

Snack:

- 1 cup yogurt

Lunch:

- Ancient Grain Pasta Salad (see recipe) with peas and fresh ricotta cheese [serving size 100 grams (3.5 ounces) uncooked pasta]
- mixed green salad with 1 Tbsp vinegar, 1 Tbsp evoo, salt and pepper to taste

Snack:

- ¼ cup nuts
- coffee or tea optional

Dinner:

- Bean Cauliflower Soup (serving size 1 soup bowl)
- Grilled Vegetables (see recipe)
- 1 slice whole grain bread
- 1 glass wine optional

Snack:

- 1 cup seasonal fruit

It is time to end your day and unwind.

Shut all electronics off 1-2 hours before bedtime.

Go through your day and think about 3 good things that have happened to you and be grateful.

Make sure that you sleep 7 to 9 hours tonight.

Find 10 minutes to stretch and meditate before going to bed.
Have a good night.

Day 19

Good morning! Start your day thinking about 3 things you are grateful for. Don't forget to dance, walk, skip, jump, meditate today.

Breakfast:

- Oatmeal, (see recipe) ¼ cup raisins, 1 tsp raw honey (serving size 1 cup cooked oatmeal)
- 1 cup mixed berries
- coffee or tea optional

Snack:

- ¼ cup of nuts

Lunch:

- Sicilian Tuna in Agrodolce (see recipe) (8 ounces)
- Orange Fennel Sicilian Salad (see recipe)

Snack:

- 1 cup yogurt
- coffee or tea optional

Dinner:

- Squash and Mushroom or Spinach Creamy Soup (see recipe) (1 soup bowl)
- Kamut Chickpea Salad or Lentil and Barley Salad (see recipes) (1 cup cooked)
- 1 slice whole wheat bread
- 1 glass wine optional

Snack:

- 1 Poached Pear (see recipe)

It is time to end your day and unwind.

Shut all electronics off 1-2 hours before bedtime.

Go through your day and think about 3 good things that have happened to you and be grateful.

Make sure that you sleep 7 to 9 hours tonight.

Find 10 minutes to stretch and meditate before going to bed.
Have a good night.

Day 20

Good morning! Start your day thinking about 3 things you are grateful for. Don't forget to dance, walk, skip, jump, meditate today.

Breakfast:

- Asparagus Frittata
- 1 glass fresh squeezed orange juice
- coffee or tea optional

Snack:

- yogurt

Lunch:

- Baked Halibut and Kalamata Olives (see recipe)
- mixed green salad

Snack:

- 1 cup seasonal fruit
- coffee or tea optional

Dinner:

- Minestrone Soup (see recipe) (1 soup bowl)
- 1 slice whole grain bread
- Steamed Broccoli di Rabe (see recipe) with 1 Tbsp EVOO and 1 clove of minced garlic

Snack:

- 2 ounces dark chocolate

It is time to end your day and unwind.

Shut all electronics off 1-2 hours before bedtime.

Go through your day and think about 3 good things that have happened to you and be grateful.

Make sure that you sleep 7 to 9 hours tonight.

Find 10 minutes to stretch and meditate before going to bed.
Have a good night.

Day 21

Good morning! Start your day thinking about 3 things you are grateful for. Don't forget to dance, walk, skip, jump, meditate today.

Breakfast:

- smoothie: 1 cup kale, 1 cup spinach, ½ cucumber, ½ pear, ½ banana, ½ cup whole milk, ½ Tbsp flax seeds, ½ Tbsp chia seeds, 1 tsp raw honey. Place all the ingredients into a blender. Purée.
- coffee or tea optional

Snack:

- ¼ cup nuts

Lunch:

- String Bean, Potato and Egg Salad (see recipe)
- Bean and Quinoa Salad (see recipe)

Snack:

- 3 ounces pecorino or Parmigiano cheese
- coffee or tea optional

Dinner:

- Free-Range Chicken Cacciatore (see recipe) (3.5 ounces)
- Sautéed Spinach (see recipe)
- 1 slice whole grain bread
- 1 glass wine optional

Snack:

- 1 cup seasonal fruit

It is time to end your day and unwind.

Shut all electronics off 1-2 hours before bedtime.

Go through your day and think about 3 good things that have happened to you and be grateful.

Make sure that you sleep 7 to 9 hours tonight.

Find 10 minutes to stretch and meditate before going to bed.
Have a good night.

CONGRATULATIONS!

YOU HAVE COMPLETED YOUR 3RD week! Take a moment to congratulate yourself and ask yourself how you are feeling. Have you enjoyed your meals? Are you feeling stronger and healthier? Do you know your farmer market by now? Can you take more steps every day?

Day 22

Good morning! Start your day thinking about 3 things you are grateful for. Don't forget to dance, walk, skip, jump, meditate today.

Breakfast:

- Creamy Farro (see recipe), ½ cup chopped mixed dry fruit, 1 tsp raw honey (1 cup cooked farro)
- 1 glass of fresh squeezed orange juice
- coffee or tea optional

Snack:

- ¼ cup nuts

Lunch:

- Ancient Grain Pasta Salad (see recipe) with cherry tomatoes or sun dry tomatoes
- mixed green salad

Snack:

- 1 cup seasonal fruit
- coffee or tea optional

Dinner:

- Fava Bean Soup (see recipe) (1 soup bowl)
- Peas and Artichoke Stew (see recipe) (1 cup cooked vegetables)
- 1 slice of whole grain bread

Snack:

- 1 cup yogurt and 1 tsp raw honey

It is time to end your day and unwind.

Shut all electronics off 1-2 hours before bedtime.

Go through your day and think about 3 good things that have happened to you and be grateful.

Make sure that you sleep 7 to 9 hours tonight.

Find 10 minutes to stretch and meditate before going to bed.
Have a good night.

Day 23

Good morning! Start your day thinking about 3 things you are grateful for. Don't forget to dance, walk, skip, jump, meditate today.

Breakfast:

- smoothie: ½ cup mixed berries, ½ banana, 1 cup spinach, 1 cup kale, ½ cup yogurt, 1½ Tbsp flax seeds, ½ Tbsp chia seeds. Place all the ingredients into a blender. Purée.
- coffee or tea optional

Snack:

- cappuccino, 1 slice whole grain bread with jam

Lunch:

- **Organic Free-Range Chicken Soup** (see recipe) (1 soup bowl)
- **Steamed Broccoli** (see recipe) with 1 Tbsp **EVOO** and fresh squeezed lemon juice, salt and pepper to taste

Snack:

- ¼ cup nuts
- coffee or tea optional

Dinner:

- Kamut Chickpea Salad (see recipe) (1 cup cooked)
- mixed green salad with 1 Tbsp vinegar and 1 Tbsp EVOO, salt and pepper to taste
- 1 glass wine optional

Snack:

- 2 ounces dark chocolate

It is time to end your day and unwind.

Shut all electronics off 1-2 hours before bedtime.

Go through your day and think about 3 good things that have happened to you and be grateful.

Make sure that you sleep 7 to 9 hours tonight.

Find 10 minutes to stretch and meditate before going to bed.
Have a good night.

Day 24

Good morning! Start your day thinking about 3 things you are grateful for. Don't forget to dance, walk, skip, jump, meditate today.

Breakfast:

- Spinach Frittata (see recipe)
- 1 slice whole grain bread
- 1 glass fresh squeezed orange juice
- coffee or tea optional

Snack:

- 1 cup yogurt

Lunch:

- Polenta (see recipe) in chicken or vegetable broth (1 cup cooked polenta)
- Sautéed Mushrooms (see recipe)
- mixed green salad with 1 Tbsp vinegar, 1 Tbsp EVOO, salt and pepper to taste

Snack:

- ¼ cup of nuts
- coffee or tea optional

Dinner:

- Pan-Seared Flounder (see recipe) (8 ounces)
- Lentil and Barley Salad (see recipe) (1 cup)
- 1 glass of wine optional

Snack:

- ½ cup whole warm milk with 1 ounce of chocolate

It is time to end your day and unwind.

Shut all electronics off 1-2 hours before bedtime.

Go through your day and think about 3 good things that have happened to you and be grateful.

Make sure that you sleep 7 to 9 hours tonight.

Find 10 minutes to stretch and meditate before going to bed.
Have a good night.

Day 25

Good morning! Start your day thinking about 3 things you are grateful for. Don't forget to dance, walk, skip, jump, meditate today.

Breakfast:
- ¼ cup Homemade Granola (see recipe) in ½ cup whole milk
- 1 cup seasonal fruit

Snack:
- 1 cup yogurt

Lunch:
- Ancient Grain Pasta Salad (see recipe) [100 grams (3.5 ounces) uncooked pasta]
- mixed green salad

Snack:
- 2 cups raw vegetables with 2 Tbsp Eggplant Spread (see recipe)
- coffee or tea optional

Dinner:

- Marinated Grilled, Free-Range Chicken (see recipe) with roasted potato (3.5 ounces)
- Steamed Cauliflower (see recipe) with 1 Tbsp EVOO and fresh squeezed lemon, salt and pepper to taste

Snack:

- ¼ cup roasted nuts sprinkled with raw cane sugar

It is time to end your day and unwind.

Shut all electronics off 1-2 hours before bedtime.

Go through your day and think about 3 good things that have happened to you and be grateful.

Make sure that you sleep 7 to 9 hours tonight.

Find 10 minutes to stretch and meditate before going to bed.
Have a good night.

Day 26

Good morning! Start your day thinking about 3 things you are grateful for. Don't forget to dance, walk, skip, jump, meditate today.

Breakfast:

- cappuccino, ½ cup whole milk
- 1 slice whole grain bread with jam
- 1 cup seasonal fruit

Snack:

- ¼ cup nuts

Lunch:

- Minestrone Soup (see recipe) (1 bowl)
- Kamut Chickpea Salad (see recipe) (1 cup cooked kamut)
- Orange Fennel Sicilian Salad (see recipe)

Snack:

- yogurt

Dinner:

- Squash and Mushroom Soup (see recipe) (one bowl)
- mixed green salad with 1 Tbsp venegar, 1 Tbsp EVOO, salt and pepper to taste
- 1 slice whole grain bread

Snack:

- 1 cup seasonal fruit

It is time to end your day and unwind.

Shut all electronics off 1-2 hours before bedtime.

Go through your day and think about 3 good things that have happened to you and be grateful.

Make sure that you sleep 7 to 9 hours tonight.

Find 10 minutes to stretch and meditate before going to bed.
Have a good night.

Day 27

Good morning! Start your day thinking about 3 things you are grateful for. Don't forget to dance, walk, skip, jump, meditate today.

Breakfast:

- 1 soft boiled egg
- 1 slice whole grain bread with jam
- 1 glass fresh squeezed orange juice

Snack:

- 1 cup yogurt

Lunch:

- Grilled Salmon (see recipe) with Salmoriglio sauce (see recipe) (8 ounces)
- Grilled Vegetables (see recipe)
- mixed green salad with 1 Tbsp vinegar, 1 Tbsp EVOO, salt and pepper to taste

Snack:

- 1 cup seasonal fruit

Dinner:

- Ancient Grain Pasta Salad with Pesto Sauce (see recipes) [100 grams (3.5 ounces) uncooked pasta, 2 Tbsp Pesto Sauce]
- Summer Tomatoes, Red Onion Salad (see recipe)
- Steamed Broccoli di Rabe (see recipe)
- 1 glass wine optional

Snack:

- ½ cup of toasted nuts sprinkled with raw cane sugar

It is time to end your day and unwind.

Shut all electronics off 1-2 hours before bedtime.

Go through your day and think about 3 good things that have happened to you and be grateful.

Make sure that you sleep 7 to 9 hours tonight.

Find 10 minutes to stretch and meditate before going to bed.
Have a good night.

Day 28

Good morning! Start your day thinking about 3 things you are grateful for. Don't forget to dance, walk, skip, jump, meditate today.

Breakfast:

- Onion, Pecorino Frittata (see recipe)
- 1 slice of whole grain bread
- 1 glass of fresh squeezed orange juice
- coffee or tea optional

Snack:

- raw vegetables with hummus

Lunch:

- Grilled Eggplants and Meatballs (see recipe)
- Bean and Quinoa Salad (see recipe) (1 cup cooked quinoa)
- mixed green salad with 1 Tbsp vinegar, 1 Tbsp EVOO, salt and pepper to taste

Snack:

- 1 cup yogurt
- coffee or tea optional

Dinner:

- Lentil and Farro Soup (see recipe) (1 cup cooked farro)
- 1 slice whole grain bread
- 3 ounces pecorino or Parmigiano cheese
- mixed green salad with 1 Tbsp vinegar, 1 Tbsp EVOO, salt and pepper to taste
- 1 glass wine optional

Snack:

- 2 ounces dark chocolate

It is time to end your day and unwind.

Shut all electronics off 1-2 hours before bedtime.

Go through your day and think about 3 good things that have happened to you and be grateful.

Make sure that you sleep 7 to 9 hours tonight.

Find 10 minutes to stretch and meditate before going to bed.
Have a good night.

Day 29

Good morning! Start your day thinking about 3 things you are grateful for. Don't forget to dance, walk, skip, jump, meditate today.

Breakfast:

- ½ cup Homemade Granola (see recipe), ½ cup of whole milk
- 1 cup seasonal fruit
- coffee or tea optional

Snack:

- ¼ cup nuts

Lunch:

- Marinated Grilled Pork Chops (3.5 ounces)
- Roasted Eggplants and Zucchini (see recipe)
- mixed green salad with 1 Tbsp vinegar, 1 Tbsp EVOO, salt and pepper to taste

Snack:

- 1 cup yogurt
- coffee or tea optional

Dinner:

- Mixed Bean Soup (see recipe) (1 soup bowl)
- 1 slice whole grain bread
- Steamed Broccoli (see recipe) with 1 Tbsp EVOO, salt and pepper to taste

Snack:

- 1 cup seasonal fruit

It is time to end your day and unwind.

Shut all electronics off 1-2 hours before bedtime.

Go through your day and think about 3 good things that have happened to you and be grateful.

Make sure that you sleep 7 to 9 hours tonight.

Find 10 minutes to stretch and meditate before going to bed.
Have a good night.

Day 30

Good morning! Start your day thinking about 3 things you are grateful for. Don't forget to dance, walk, skip, jump, meditate today.

Breakfast:
- Spinach Frittata (see recipe)
- 1 slice whole grain bread
- 1 glass fresh squeezed orange juice
- coffee or tea optional

Snack:
- 1 cup yogurt

Lunch:
- Ancient Grain Pasta Salad with Classic Tomato Sauce (see recipes) [100 grams (3.5 ounces) uncooked pasta, 5 Tbsp Classic Tomato Sauce (see recipe)]
- mixed green salad with 1 Tbsp vinegar, 1 Tbsp EVOO, salt and pepper to taste

Snack:
- ¼ cup nuts
- coffee or tea optional

Dinner:

- Branzino (see recipe) with Salmoriglio sauce (see recipe) (8 ounces)
- Lentil and Barley Salad (see recipe) (1 cup)
- Orange, Fennel Sicilian Salad (see recipe)

Snack:

- 1 cup seasonal fruit

It is time to end your day and unwind.

Shut all electronics off **1-2** hours before bedtime.

Go through your day and think about **3** good things that have happened to you and be grateful.

Make sure that you sleep **7** to **9** hours tonight.

Find **10** minutes to stretch and meditate before going to bed.
Have a good night.

CONGRATULATIONS!

You have completed your 30 day plan! Take a moment to congratulate yourself and observe how you are feeling today a month after you started this journey! You have connected with your ancestors, the ones that have come to occupied Sicily and left behind with their DNA a piece of their culinary history. Hopefully this connection has helped you to feel healthier, stronger and happier.

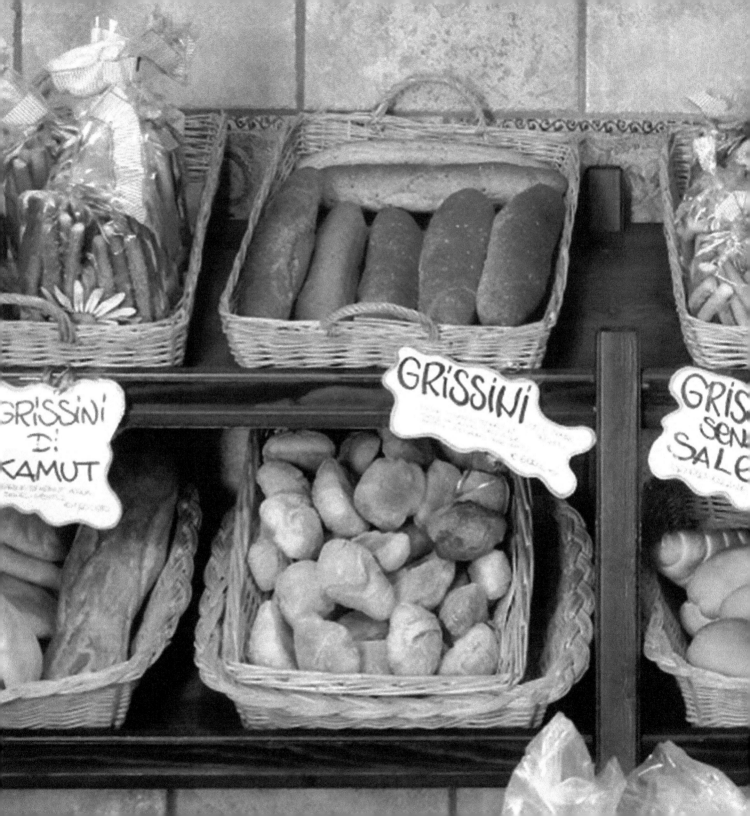

Chapter 16

RECIPES FOR THE SICILIAN DIET

How to eat your way to good health

Breakfast Recipes

Homemade Granola (serves 10)

- ⅓ cup honey
- ¼ cup maple syrup
- 5 cups of oats
- 2 cups mixed chopped nuts
- 2 cups mixed chopped dried fruit (i.e.: figs, cranberries, raisins, dates, apricot)
- 1 cup canola oil (optional) will help the granola to stick together but will add more monounsaturated fat.

Turn the oven to 325° F. Place the honey in a glass container with cup of water and melt in the microwave for 10 seconds. Whisk the maple syrup and honey in a large bowl, mix the oats with the chopped nuts until they are thoroughly covered. Spray a baking pan with canola oil and spread the mixed oats evenly. Bake at 350° F. for 40 minutes mixing it with a wooden or metal spoon every 15 min. When done, add the dried fruit, mix well. Bring to room temperature. Serve. Can be stored in the refrigerator up to 3 weeks.

Bulgur Wheat with Roasted Almonds (serves 2)

- ½ cup bulgur wheat
- ¼ cup roasted almonds
- 1 Tbsp organic unrefined sugar
- ½ tsp cinnamon
- ½ cup berries
- organic orange zest

Cook the bulgur wheat in 1 cup of water. The grain is ready when all the water is absorbed. Toast the almonds and sugar in a pan stirring often until golden. Mix the almonds and all other ingredients together. Serve.

Oatmeal, Raisin (serves 2)

(serving size 1 cup of cooked oatmeal)

- 1 cup oatmeal
- ½ cup water
- ½ cup whole milk
- salt to taste
- ½ chopped apple
- ½ cup toasted walnuts
- 1 tsp maple syrup
- ½ cup raisins

Cook 1 cup oatmeal in ½ cup water and half cup of milk until creamy, add salt, apple, walnut, maple syrup and ½ cup raisins and cook for 3 minutes. Serve.

Creamy Farro with Roasted Grapes (serves 2)

- 1 cup farro or kamut
- 1 cup milk
- 1 piece cinnamon stick
- pinch of salt to taste
- 2 cups grapes (or plums or pear or apple)
- 1 Tbsp honey or 1 Tbsp maple syrup
- 1 Tbsp water
- ½ tsp vanilla extract
- ground cinnamon (optional)

Cook the farro in 1 cup of water and 1 cup of milk with the cinnamon stick and salt. Preheat the oven to broiler, spread the grapes over a baking sheet. Place the honey in a microwavable bowl with **1** Tbsp of water and place in the microwave for 10 seconds, mix the honey and water and sprinkle over the grapes. Broil for 6 minutes. Add grapes, vanilla extract, and cook for 2 minutes. Sprinkle with ground cinnamon (optional). Serve.

Creamy Farro (serves 2)

- 1 cup farro
- 1 cup water
- 1 cup milk
- 1 stick cinnamon
- 1 pinch salt
- 1 tsp vanilla extract

Cook the farro in 1 cup of water and 1 cup of milk with the cinnamon stick and salt at medium-low heat. The farro is ready when all the liquid is absorbed. Add the vanilla extract and mix. Serve.

Spinach Frittata (serves 2)

(Spinach can be substituted with ½ cup cooked asparagus or ½ cup cooked broccoli or ½ cup sautéed mushrooms or ½ cup caramelized onions.)

- 2 free-range organic eggs
- salt and pepper to taste
- 1 Tbsp Parmesan or pecorino cheese
- 1 cup chopped organic baby spinach
- ½ Tbsp EVOO

In a small bowl whisk the eggs, add salt and pepper and whisk again. Add the Parmesan cheese and spinach and mix. Place the EVOO in a small omelette pan, when the oil is hot add the egg mixture, lower the heat to medium for 4 minutes lifting the sides with a fork. When the egg is set to one side place a flat dish over the skillet and flip the frittata onto the dish then quickly back into the skillet and cook until the egg is fully set (4 minutes).

For the onion frittata: sauté one Vidalia onion finely chopped in the omelette pan with ½ Tbsp EVOO, after 5 minutes add salt and pepper. Add ½ cup of water and cook for 10 minutes at low heat. Let the onion cool down for a few minutes then add it to the egg mixture. Follow the directions for the Spinach Frittata.

Asparagus Frittata (serves 2)

- **20 asparagus stalks**
- **4 free-range eggs or 6 egg whites**
- **1 Tbsp of parmigiano cheese**
- **salt and pepper to taste**
- **½ Tbsp EVOO**

Wash the asparagus and remove the tough part of the stem. Boil or steam the asparagus for 5 minutes, then cut in small pieces.

Beat the eggs with cheese, salt and pepper.

Add the asparagus to the cheese batter.

Place the EVOO in a small non-stick skillet and let the oil coat the skillet. When the oil is hot but not burning, add the egg batter. Cook on one side until the batter lifts with a fork on all sides. Place a large dish over the frittata, flip the frittata over the dish and place the top side back onto the skillet and cook until the egg batter is firm. Serve.

Onion, Pecorino Frittata (serves 2)

- **1 medium onion**
- **1 Tbsp EVOO**
- **salt and pepper to taste**
- **4 free-range eggs or 6 egg whites**
- **2 Tbsp freshly grated pecorino cheese**

Chop the onion into small sizes.

Place ½ of the olive oil in a small non-stick skillet, add the onion and cook at low medium-heat for 8 minutes with a lid on, stirring occasionally. Add pepper and salt to the onion while cooking. (Continued on next page.)

Beat the eggs with the cheese. Remove the onion from the stove and incorporate into the egg batter.

Wipe the skillet with a paper towel and place the rest of the olive oil onto the skillet.

Turn the heat to medium-high. Let the oil coat the skillet. When the oil is hot but not burning, add the egg batter.

Cook on one side until the batter lifts with a fork on all sides.

Place a large dish over the frittata, flip the frittata over the dish and place the top side back onto the skillet and cook until the egg batter is firm. Serve.

Grits (stone-ground whole grain, available by Bob's Red Mill) and Greek yogurt (serves 2)

- 1 cup stone-ground grits
- 2 cups water
- ½ cup Greek yogurt
- 1 tsp manuka honey (any raw honey is a good substitute)
- ¼ cup organic orange peel
- ¼ cup raisins

Cook 1 cup grits in 2 cups of water. The grits will be ready when the water is absorbed.

Let the grits cool then add yogurt, honey, orange peel and raisins. Serving size is 1 cup cooked grits.

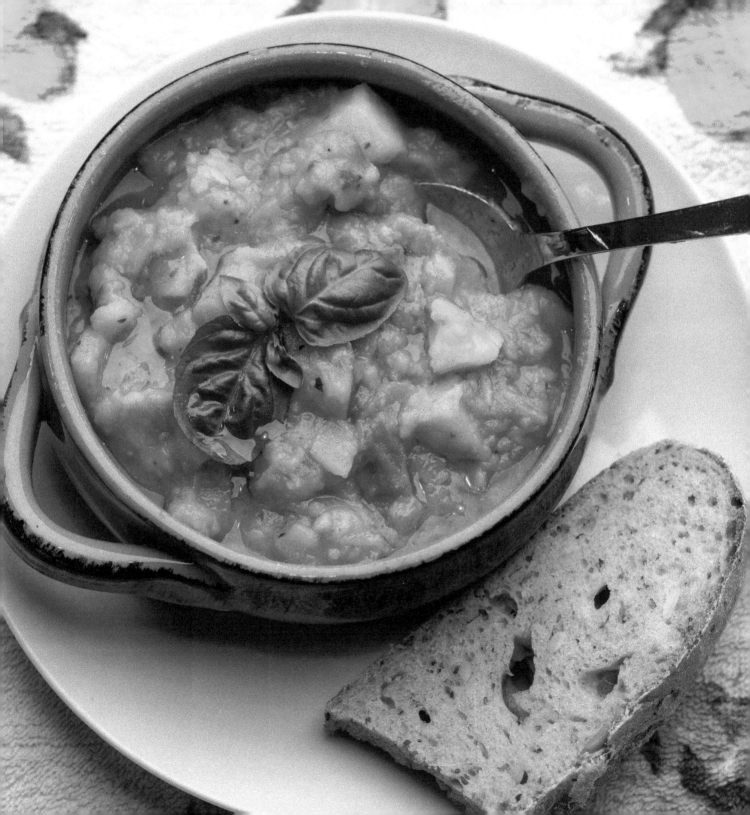

Soups

Minestrone (serves 2)

- 1 yellow onion, chopped
- 1 Tbsp EVOO
- salt, pepper to taste (chopped fresh basil and chopped fresh garlic optional.)
- 1 tomato, diced
- 1 potato, diced
- 2 celery stalks, chopped
- 2 zucchini, diced
- 1 carrot, diced
- 1 cup water

Sauté the chopped onion in olive oil at low-medium heat until the onion is soft and lightly brown, add salt and pepper half way.

Add the chopped vegetables and stir for 5 minutes, add water and cover. Cook at low-medium heat for 30 minutes. Place half of the cooked vegetables in a blender or use a hand mixer to purée half of the vegetables for a creamier taste (optional). Add chopped fresh basil and garlic (optional). Serve hot.

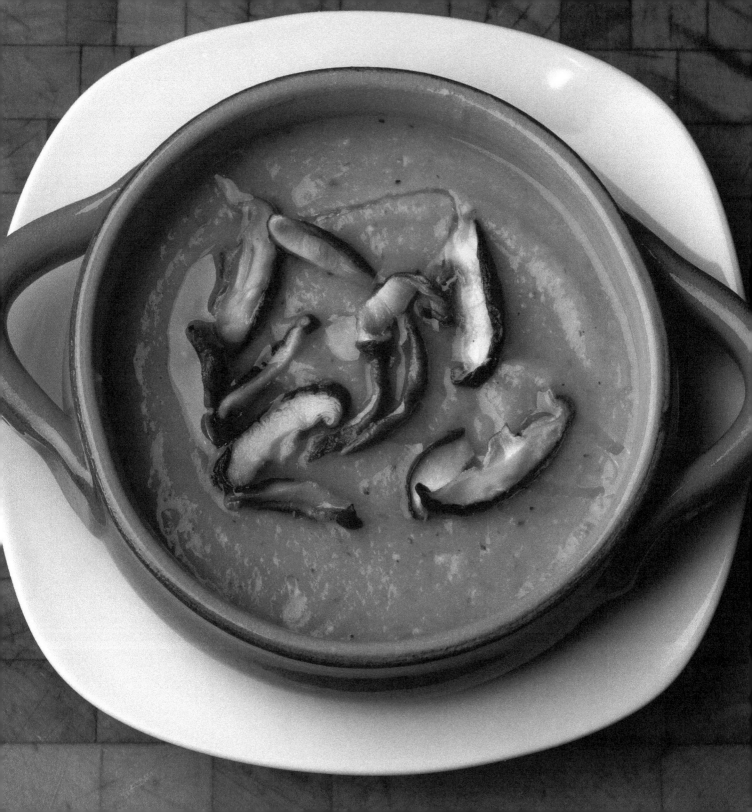

Squash and Mushroom Soup (serves 2)

- 1 medium butternut squash halved, seeds removed
- 2 ½ Tbsp EVOO
- salt and pepper to taste
- 5 cups vegetable broth
- 1 large onion, chopped
- 2 cups mixed chopped mushrooms

Place the squash on a baking pan, sprinkle with 2 Tbsp olive oil, salt and pepper and bake in a 350° F. oven for 45 minutes or till a fork can push through the flesh without resistance.

Let it cool for a few minutes then scrape the flesh and place it into a bowl.

Bring the broth to boil, add the chopped onion, 1 cup of mushrooms and the squash. Bring it to a low simmer and cook for 15 minutes.

Sauté the remaining mushrooms in a small skillet with ½ Tbsp EVOO

Place the soup in a blender or food processor and blend until creamy. Bring back to the pot and add the sautéed mushrooms. Stir and serve hot.

Lentil Soup (serves 3)

- 1 ½ cup of lentils
- 2 stalks celery, chopped
- 1 tomato, diced
- 1 onion, chopped
- 1 carrot, diced
- salt and pepper to taste
- 2 Tbsp EVOO

Place the lentils and vegetables in a pot, cover with water. Add salt and bring to a boil. Lower the heat to low to maintain a soft boil for 45 minutes. Add olive oil, serve hot.

Mixed Bean Soup or Cauliflower Bean Soup (serves 4)

- 2 cups of mixed dry beans
- 2 stalks celery, chopped
- 1 tomato, diced
- 1 onion, chopped
- 1 carrot, diced
- salt and pepper to taste
- 2 Tbsp EVOO
- 1 small cauliflower head (for Cauliflower Bean Soup)

Soak the beans overnight in a large pot. Drain and rinse. Place the beans and vegetables in a pot, cover with water. Add salt and bring to the boil. Lower the heat to low to maintain a soft boil for 45 minutes. Add olive oil, serve hot. For Cauliflower Bean Soup, cut the cauliflower stem. Cut the florets and with a sharp knife, remove the tougher outer layer of the floret stems. Add the cauliflower florets to the Bean Soup after cooking the beans for 35 minutes so the cauliflower cooks with the beans for 10 minutes. Serve hot.

Organic Free-Range Chicken Soup (serves 4)

- 1 whole organic free-range chicken
- 3 organic free-range bones (lamb, beef, veal, chicken back, neck)
- 2 stalks celery, chopped
- 1 tomato, diced
- 1 large onion, chopped
- 1 carrot, diced
- 1 cup fresh parsley
- salt and pepper to taste

Place the chicken, bones, vegetables, salt and pepper in a large pot. Cover with water and bring to the boil. Lower the heat and cook maintaining a soft boil for 90 minutes. Serve hot.

Chickpea Soup (serves 4)

- 1 onion, chopped
- 1 carrot, chopped
- 1 stalk celery, chopped
- 1 leek, chopped
- 2 Tbsp EVOO
- 2 cups of dry chickpeas soaked overnight
- 6 cups vegetable broth or water
- 2 cups spinach
- salt and pepper to taste

Sauté the chopped onion, carrot, celery and leek in one Tbsp of olive oil until golden and soft. Add the drained chickpeas and stir well into the sautéed vegetables. Add the broth and cook at a low simmer for 2 hours. Add the spinach and cook for 5 minutes. If you like your soups creamier, place half of the soaked chickpeas in a blender then mix it back into the soup. Add the remaining Tbsp of olive oil and serve hot.

Fava Bean, Chicoria (Chicory) or Spinach Creamy Soup (serves 2)

- 4 cups water
- salt to taste
- 1 large onion, chopped
- 2 cups of shelled fava beans soaked overnight
- 2 cups of spinach or 1 head of cicoria
- 2 Tbsp EVOO

Place 4 cups of water in a medium skillet, add salt, chopped onion and fava beans and cook for ½ hour. Add the spinach or chicoria and cook for 15 minutes. Place the soup in a blender until creamy, return to the stove to keep hot before serving. Add olive oil and serve hot.

Lentil and Farro Soup (serves 2)

- 2 cups lentil
- 1 cup farro
- 1 carrot, chopped
- 1 onion, chopped
- 1 celery stalk, chopped
- 1 tomato, diced
- salt and pepper to taste
- 2 Tbsp EVOO

Place all ingredients except olive oil, salt and pepper in a large pot. Cover with water standing 1 inch above the ingredients. Cook at medium heat with the lid on for 30 minutes. You can blend ⅓ of the soup for extra creaminess if you want. Add olive oil, salt and pepper. Serve hot.

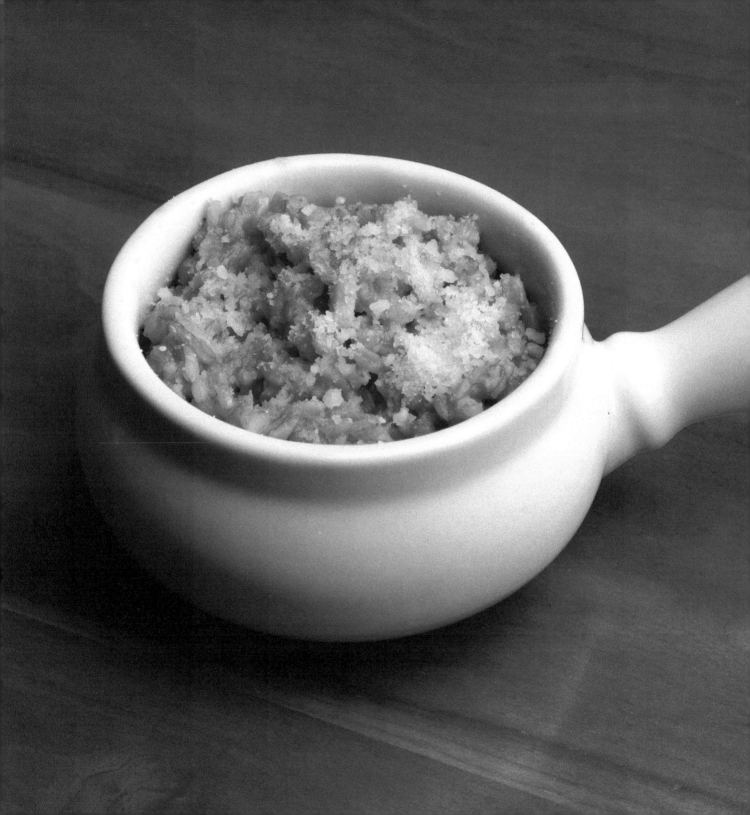

Farro Parmesan Risotto (serves 2)

- 1 Tbsp EVOO
- 1 large onion, chopped
- salt to taste
- 1 cup of farro soaked overnight
- 2 cups of chicken or vegetable broth
- 2 Tbsp Parmesan cheese

Place the olive oil in a medium-size pot. Add the onion and cook until golden and soft. Add salt. Add the farro and stir well into the onion. Add the chicken broth. Cover the pot and cook at a low simmer until all the broth is absorbed. Stir the Parmesan cheese. Keep it covered for 5 minutes and serve hot.

Polenta (1 cup cooked polenta)

- 5 cups vegetarian broth or chicken broth
- 1 cup stone-ground whole grain grits
- 1 Tbsp butter
- 2 Tbsp Parmesan cheese

Bring the broth to boil in a medium-size pot. When the broth is simmering, slowly add the polenta (grits) a little at the time, stirring continuously with a wooden spoon. Continue to stir often for 15 minutes. Add the butter and Parmesan cheese and serve hot.

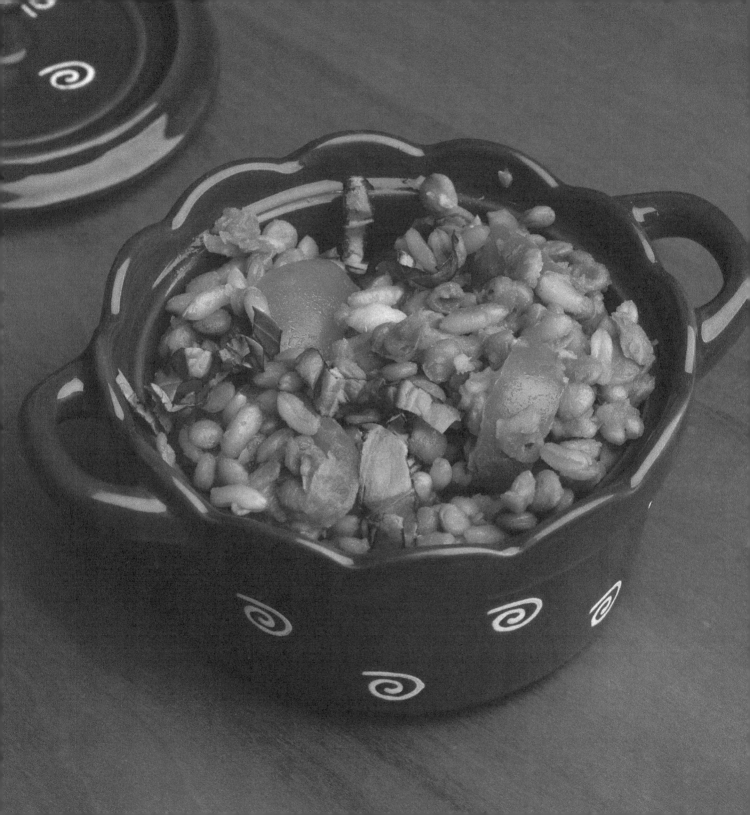

Salads

Lentil and Barley Salad (serves 4)

- 1 cup of whole barley
- 1 cup of lentils
- 1 bay leaf
- ½ red onion sliced very thin
- 1 clove garlic, minced
- 1 yellow pepper sliced very thin
- 1 cup cherry tomatoes, halved
- 1 Tbsp balsamic or red wine vinegar
- 1 Tbsp apple cider vinegar
- 1 Tbsp EVOO
- 1 cup chopped fresh parsley
- salt and pepper to taste

Cook the barley in 2 ½ cups of salted water for 40 or 50 minutes. The barley will be ready when most of the water is absorbed and the grain is tender. Drain and place in a large bowl. Cook the lentils in 3 cups of salted water and bay leaf for 40 minutes. Drain the lentils and discard the bay leaf. Mix the lentils with the barley, add the onion, garlic, pepper, tomato, vinegars and olive oil. Before serving mix in the parsley. Serve cold.

Cannellini Bean and Red Onion Salad (serves 2)

- 1 lb organic canned cannellini beans, drained
- 1 red onion, sliced very thin
- 1 Tbsp EVOO
- 1 Tbsp vinegar
- salt and pepper to taste
- cherry tomatoes (optional)

Mix all the ingredients together, serve cold.

Ancient Grain Pasta Salad (serves 2)

- 1 Tbsp EVOO
- 1 Tbsp vinegar
- salt and red pepper to taste
- ½ red onion cut very thin
- ½ cup of pitted kalamata olives
- 1 cup halved cherry tomatoes
- ½ lb ancient grain or whole grain pasta (fusilli or bow tie shape is best)
- 1 Tbsp of grated pecorino cheese optional

Marinate the olive oil, vinegar, salt and red pepper, onion, kalamata olives and cherry tomatoes in a bowl for 2 or more hours. Bring a pot of salted water to a boil. Add the pasta. Following the box instructions cook the pasta al dente. Drain well and place the pasta in the bowl with the marinated olives and tomatoes. Mix well and serve cold. Add pecorino cheese, optional.

Bulgur Wheat, Lentil, Olive Salad (serves 2)

- 1 cup bulgur wheat
- 2 cups water
- 1 cup lentils
- 4 cups water
- 1 bay leaf, optional
- ½ cup kalamata olives, finely chopped
- 1 small red onion, finely chopped
- 2 Tbsp EVOO
- 2 Tbsp red wine vinegar
- salt and pepper to taste

Cook the bulgur wheat in a small pot with 2 cups of water for 10 minutes or until the water is absorbed.

Cook the lentils for 25 minutes in a small pot with 4 cups of salted water and one bay leaf. Remove the bay leaf and excessive water from the lentils.

Place all ingredients in a bowl and serve warm or cold.

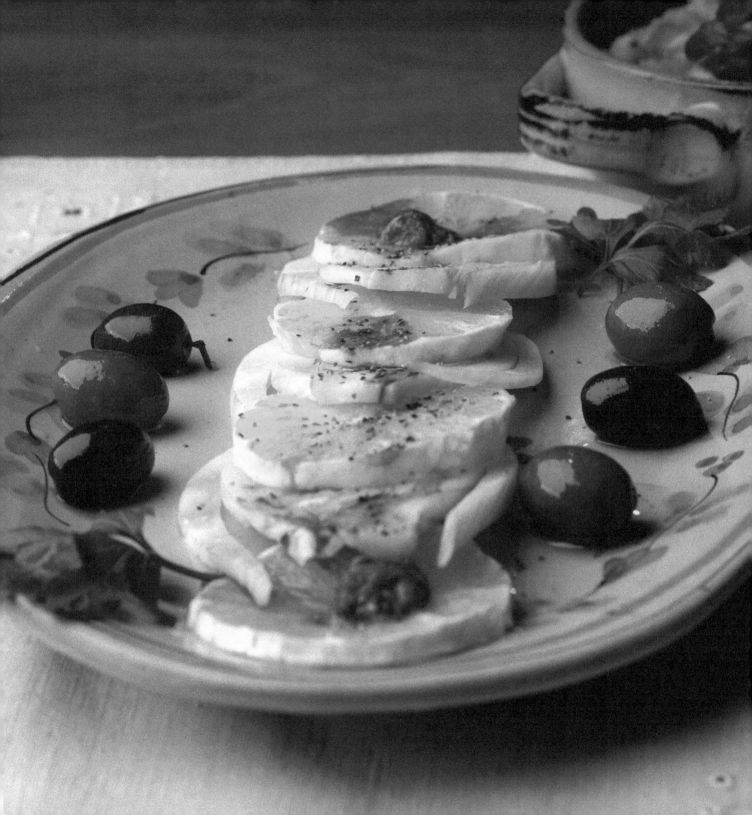

Orange, Fennel Sicilian Salad (serves 2)

Orange salad is a typical Sicilian salad (Catania), which uses several of the island's prime materials such as anchovies, oranges, and olive oil.
The Arabs imported the orange trees from the orient. In some parts of Sicily the oranges are still called "portuallu" because they came from Europe through Portugal.

This salad uses salted fish. Sicily produces the largest variety of salted fish, more than any other Italian region. Salt has always been readily available on the island and its seas were rich in fish. Salting fish allowed to conserve it during the months where fishing is scarce.

- 1 orange, large
- 1 fennel bulb
- 6 kalamata olives
- 2 anchovies (optional)
- salt and pepper to taste
- 1 Tbsp red wine vinegar
- 1 Tbsp EVOO

Peel the orange and cut it in very thin slices. Wash and cut the fennel in very thin slices and place on the serving plate alternating orange and fennel slices. Add the olives and anchovies. Sprinkle salt and pepper, vinegar and EVOO. Serve.

Kamut Chickpea Salad (serves 4)

- 1 cup kamut soaked overnight

- 2 cups water, salted to taste

- 1 organic 13-ounce canned chickpea or 1 cup chickpeas soaked overnight

- 2 Tbsp EVOO

- 2 Tbsp vinegar

- 1 red onion sliced very thin

- 15 cherry tomatoes, halved

- salt and pepper to taste

- fresh basil, chopped (optional)

Cook the kamut in 2 cups of salted water for 50 minutes (low simmer), add the canned chickpeas. If you use the soaked dry chickpeas cook them in 3 cups of salted water with one bay leaf for 50 minutes then drain. Mix the chickpeas and kamut. Add oil, vinegar, onion, cherry tomatoes, salt, pepper and fresh basil. Serve cold.

Arugula, Avocado Salad (serves 2)

- 1 Tbsp EVOO
- 1 Tbsp vinegar
- salt and pepper to taste
- 4 cups of washed arugula
- 1 peeled and chopped avocado
- ½ cup toasted nuts
- 2 ounces very thinly sliced Parmesan cheese

Whisk olive oil, vinegar, salt and pepper. Add arugula, avocado, toasted nuts, Parmesan cheese, and mix. Serve.

Summer Tomatoes, Red Onion Salad (Very good on toasted bread)

- 2 tomatoes, large
- ½ red onion sliced very thin
- salt and pepper to taste
- 1 Tbsp EVOO
- dry oregano

Slice the tomatoes, add sliced onion, salt, pepper and EVOO, sprinkle with oregano. Serve.

Bulgur Wheat, Lentil, Olive Salad (serves 2)

- 1 cup bulgur wheat
- 2 cups water
- 1 cup lentils
- 4 cups water, lightly salted to taste
- 1 bay leaf (optional)
- ½ cup kalamata olives, finely chopped
- 1 red onion, small, finely chopped
- 2 Tbsp EVOO
- 2 Tbsp red wine vinegar
- salt and pepper to taste

Cook the bulgur wheat in a small pot with 2 cups of water for 10 minutes or until the water is absorbed.

Cook the lentils for 25 minutes in a small pot with 4 cups of lightly salted water and one leaf of bay leaf. Remove the bay leaf and excessive water from the lentils.

Place all ingredients in a bowl and serve warm or cold.

Bean and Quinoa Salad (serves 2)

(Farro can be used instead of quinoa.)

- 1 cup of organic cannellini beans or any bean of your choice soaked overnight.
- 4 cups water, salted to taste
- 1 bay leaf (optional)
- ½ cup quinoa or farro
- 1 cup water
- 1 red onion, small, thinly sliced
- 1 cup cherry tomatoes
- 1 cup fresh basil
- 2 Tbsp EVOO
- 2 Tbsp red wine vinegar
- salt and pepper to taste

Rinse the soaked beans and cook, with lid on, in a medium pot with 4 cups of salted water and bay leaf for 2 hours.

Cook the quinoa in a small pot with 1 cup of water until the water is absorbed. If using farro, cook it for 20 minutes.

Cut the cherry tomatoes in halves to allow for their juice to flavor the salad.

Remove the excessive water from the beans, add all the ingredients in a bowl and mix.

Serve warm or cold.

String Bean, Potato and Egg Salad (Farro can be used instead of quinoa.) (serves 2)

- 3 cups string beans
- 2 potatoes, small
- 2 free-range, hard boiled eggs
- 2 Tbsp EVOO
- 1 Tbsp white wine vinegar (optional)
- salt and pepper to taste

Wash and trim the string beans.

Peel and dice the potatoes.

Place the potatoes and beans onto a steamer with 1 inch of water. Steam until a fork can enter the potato flesh without resistance.

Peel the eggs and slice in quarters.

Place beans, potatoes and eggs in a bowl. Add oil, vinegar, salt and pepper. Toss. Serve.

Dressing for Mixed Green Salad with Cherry Tomatoes

- ½ small red onion, thinly sliced
- 1 Tbsp EVOO
- 1 Tbsp balsamic vinegar
- salt to taste

Combine all ingredients in a mixing bowl or glass jar.

Side dishes

Roasted Peppers (serves 3)

- **4 peppers, large, preferably of different colors**
- **1 Tbsp freshly squeezed lemon juice**
- **1 Tbsp EVOO**
- **1 clove garlic, minced**
- **salt and pepper to taste**

Wash the peppers and dry them. Place them on a hot grill, place a cover to keep the moisture. (You can roast the peppers in a convection oven at 400° F. for 30 minutes.) With tongs turn the peppers every few minutes until all the pepper skin is blistered. Turn the stove off and keep the peppers covered for ½ hour until they are ready to peel. When not too hot to touch, with your fingers, pull the peppers in long thin slices and place on coriander for 10 minutes. Place on a serving bowl and add lemon, oil, garlic, salt and pepper.

Roasted Eggplants and Zucchini (serves 2)

- 2 zucchini sliced in thin longitudinal strips
- 2 eggplant sliced in thin longitudinal strips
- 2 Tbsp EVOO
- 2 Tbsp vinegar
- 2 cloves garlic, minced
- salt and pepper to taste
- chopped fresh mint (optional)

Place the zucchini and eggplants on a hot grill. Turn each slice once after 5 minutes. Place one layer of the roasted vegetables on a rectangular glass container. Place the olive oil, vinegar, garlic, salt, pepper and mint in a glass container and whisk. With a spoon sprinkle the condiment over the vegetables and form another layer and keep going until all the ingredients are used. Serve hot.

Grilled Eggplants and Meatballs (serves 2)

- 1 eggplant, large
- ½ cup bread crumbs
- 6 ounces grass-fed ground beef
- 2 Tbsp pecorino cheese
- 1 egg or 2 egg whites, beaten
- salt and pepper to taste
- ½ cup chopped fresh mint or parsley
- 2 garlic gloves, minced
- salt and pepper to taste

Make a cut with a knife on the eggplant flesh to open the skin or poke with a fork several times to prevent the eggplant from bursting in the oven. Place onto parchment paper.

Bake the eggplant at 400° F. for 20 minutes in a preheated oven or until the eggplant is soft. Let it cool.

Scoop the flesh out of the eggplant and place in a colander for 10 minutes to eliminate the water.

Place the eggplant in a bowl with the bread crumbs to absorb more of the water. Add all other ingredients and mix with your fingers.

Make small balls and flatten them a little. Place them on a hot stove-top grill or barbecue and grill 3 minutes per side. Serve hot.

Sautéed Spinach (serves 2)

- ½ cup water
- salt to taste
- 8 cups organic spinach
- 1 Tbsp EVOO
- 1 clove garlic
- red pepper flakes (optional)

Place ½ cup water in a large pot with salt. Place spinach in the pot and cook for 5 minutes. Drain. Place the oil and garlic on a skillet at medium heat or until the garlic is golden. Add the red pepper flakes and sauté the spinach for 3 minutes at medium heat. Serve hot.

Sautéed Mushrooms (serves 2) (Mushrooms are nutrient packed, immune boosting and cancer fighting food.)

- 4 cups mixed mushrooms (shiitake, chanterelle, oyster, etc.)
- 1 Tbsp EVOO
- 1 clove garlic, minced
- red pepper flakes to taste (optional)
- salt to taste
- ½ cup fresh chopped parsley

Wash the mushrooms and rinse in a salad spinner. Chop the mushrooms.

Place the EVOO, garlic, red pepper and salt in a skillet. Sauté the garlic at medium heat until golden brown. Add the mushrooms and turn the heat to high. Cook for 5 minutes stirring frequently. Place on a serving plate and add the fresh parsley.

Grilled Vegetables (serves 2)

- **1 large eggplant**
- **2 zucchini**
- **6 Tbsp EVOO**
- **6 Tbsp red wine vinegar**
- **2 gloves garlic, thinly sliced**
- **salt and red pepper to taste**
- **½ cup fresh mint, chopped**

Peel the skin from the vegetables (optional). You can grill the vegetables with skin on especially if organic and in season.

Cut the vegetables into 1-inch horizontal or vertical slices.

Place the slices onto a hot stove top or barbecue grill. Flip after 2 minutes or when grill marks are visible. Grill for 2 more minutes.

Prepare the marinade in a bowl with olive oil, vinegar, garlic, salt, red pepper, and mint.

Place one layer of grilled vegetables onto a serving dish. Sprinkle with 1 Tbsp of the marinade and keep on placing new layers and marinade. Serve.

It can be stored in the refrigerator for 5 days.

Steamed Cauliflower or Steamed Broccoli or Steamed Broccoli di Rabe (serves 2)

- 1 small cauliflower head or 1 bunch of broccoli or broccoli di rabe
- 2 Tbsp EVOO
- salt and pepper to taste
- 2 Tbsp freshly squeezed lemon juice (optional)

Cut the large stem and break the crown into smaller florets. Peel and discard the outer skin of the stem.

Bring the steamer water to boil (1-inch of water in the sauce pan). If you do not have a steamer you can place the vegetables directly onto the boiling water.

Steam or boil for 7 minutes. Dress with olive oil, salt, pepper, and freshly squeezed lemon juice.

Peas and Artichoke Stew (serves 2)

- **1 Tbsp EVOO**
- **1 small onion**
- **salt and pepper to taste**
- **1 cup frozen artichoke hearts**
- **2 cups frozen or fresh peas**
- **½ cup chopped fresh parsley**

Place the EVOO in a small skillet or small Dutch oven. Turn the heat to medium and add the chopped onion. Sauté until the onion is soft and golden. Add salt and pepper and cook for few more minutes. Add the vegetables and ½ cup of water. Cook covered stirring occasionally for 15 minutes. Add fresh parsley and serve warm.

Wild Rice and Parmigiano Cheese (serves 2)

- **1 cup of organic wild rice**
- **3 cups water, salted to taste**
- **2 Tbsp of parmigiano cheese**
- **salt and pepper to taste**
- **1 Tbsp EVOO**

Place the rice in a small pot with 3 cups of salted water.
Cook the wild rice for 20 minutes or until the water has been absorbed.
Add cheese, salt, pepper and olive oil while the rice is hot (for best melt). Incorporate the cheese, stir. Place a lid on the pot and let it sit for five minutes before serving.

Snacks

Poached Pears (Serves 4)

- 1 ⅛ cup red wine
- .82 cup water
- 1 cup sugar, unrefined
- 1 cinnamon stick
- 2 gloves
- 4 bosc pears

Place the wine, water, sugar, cinnamon and cloves in a medium pot and bring to a boil. Add the pears standing up. Bring to a simmer and cover for 30 minutes. The pears should be ready when you can insert a toothpick with ease. Remove the pears and reduce the wine to a syrup.

Serve warm with one Tbsp of syrup over each pear.

Condiments

Salmoriglio

Perfect match for grilled fish!

- 2 Tbsp EVOO
- 2 Tbsp fresh lemon juice
- salt and pepper to taste
- 1 clove garlic, minced
- ¼ cup chopped fresh parsley

Marinade for grilled meat or chicken. Combine all ingredients in a bowl. Mix. Keep the meat in the marinade for 2 hours before grilling.

Homemade Mayonnaise

- 1 whole egg
- 1 yolk
- 1 Tbsp white vinegar
- ½ fresh squeezed lemon
- salt to taste
- 1 cup canola oil

In a blender or food processor place the egg and yolk. Pulsate 4 times. Add the vinegar, lemon, and salt. Pulsate twice. Start a slow continuous stream of oil and turn the blender on until all the oil is finished. You can add 1 Tbsp of mustard to the mayonnaise for meats or eggs; you can add 1 Tbsp of capers for fish.

Eggplant Spread

- **1 large hard eggplant**
- **1 Tbsp EVOO**
- **2 Tbsp wine vinegar**
- **salt, pepper, and red pepper flakes to taste**
- **1 clove garlic, minced**

Place the eggplant on a baking dish. Cut through one side with a sharp knife to prevent the eggplant from exploding in the oven. Bake in a 400° F. oven for 45 minutes or until the eggplant is soft to the touch. Scrape the flesh and place into a bowl, mash it with a fork, add oil, vinegar, salt and pepper, and garlic. Mix well.

Sauces

Classic Tomato Sauce (3 Tbsp of sauce for one pasta portion)

- 2 Tbsp EVOO
- 1 large onion, chopped
- 2 cloves garlic
- 2 cans San Marzano tomatoes

Place the oil on a medium-size pot and turn the heat to medium. Add the onion and garlic. Let it cook until golden brown stirring occasionally. Add salt half way through. Purée the tomatoes in a blender or food processor. Add the puréed tomatoes to the onion and cook for 45 minutes at a low simmer. Serve.

Pesto Sauce

- 2 cups fresh basil leaves
- 2 garlic cloves
- salt, red pepper flakes (optional)
- ¼ cup roasted pine nuts (walnuts or almonds are good alternatives)
- ½ cup EVOO
- 1 Tbsp of Parmesan cheese (optional)
- 1 Tbsp of pecorino cheese (optional)

Place the basil, garlic, salt, and nuts in a blender or food processor. With the power on let a continuous stream of olive oil through the top. Add cheeses if desired.

For a green pesto you can blanch the basil leaves in hot water for 10 seconds, then shock it in icy water, then dry or you can add ½ cup of fresh parsley.

Simple Cherry Tomato and Sun Dried Tomato Sauce

- 2 cloves garlic, chopped
- 1 Tbsp EVOO
- 2 cups of cherry tomatoes cut in halves
- 2 sun dried tomatoes, minced
- salt and red pepper flakes to taste

Sauté the garlic in olive oil until golden brown. Add the cherry tomatoes and sun dried tomatoes. Cook for 7 minutes at medium-high heat stirring often.

Broccoli and Cauliflower Pasta Sauce (serves 2)

- 1 broccoli head
- ¼ cauliflower head
- 2 Tbsp EVOO
- 1 garlic clove, chopped
- salt to taste
- red pepper flakes (optional)
- 1 Tbsp of pecorino cheese

Wash and cut broccoli and cauliflower. Steam them for 8 minutes.

Place EVOO, garlic, salt and red pepper in a skillet and sauté at medium heat until golden brown. Add the broccoli and cauliflower and sauté for 10 minutes stirring often.

(Suggestion)

Cook ½ lb of ancient grain pasta al dente, drain but save ½ cup of pasta water to add to the sauce. Pour the pasta into the skillet with the sautéed vegetables and turn the heat to medium, add the cheese and stir for few minutes. Serve hot.

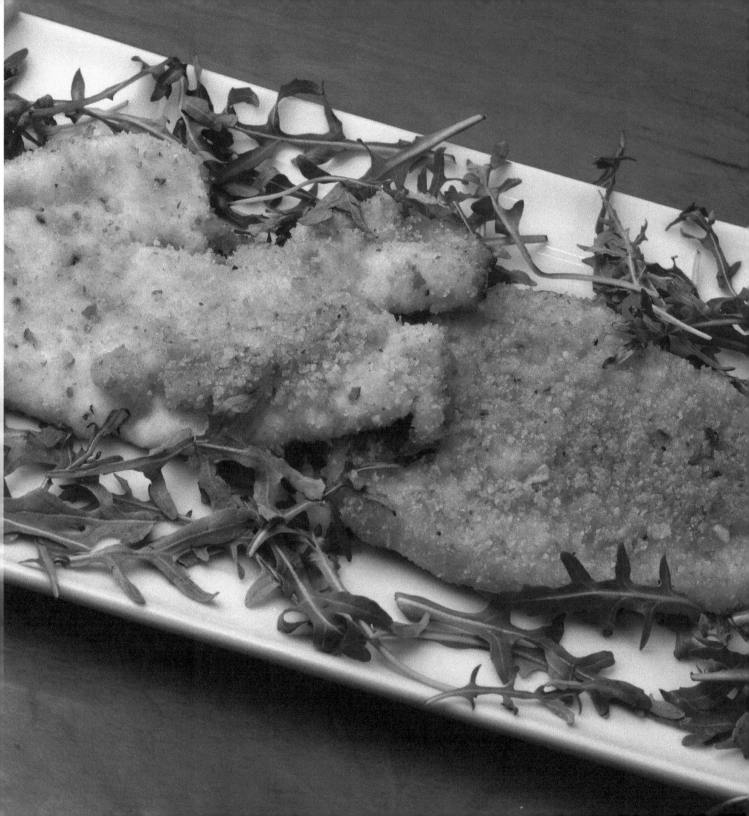

Fish

Branzino (serves 2)

- **2 branzino fillets or if you feel brave, try to steam the whole branzino**
- **½ cup white wine**
- **4 Tbsp Salmoriglio sauce (see recipe)**

Steam the branzino in ½ inch of water and white wine for 8 minutes.

If you were brave enough to cook the whole branzino, remove the head but remember to remove the cheek meat from the head. Remove the skin and the bones, sprinkle with Salmoriglio sauce and enjoy it.

Pan-Seared Flounder (serves 2)

- **2 Tbsp semolina flour**
- **2 Tbsp all-purpose flour**
- **salt and pepper to taste**
- **8 ounces flounder fillets**
- **2 Tbsp canola oil**
- **fresh lemon juice (optional)**

Place the flours, salt, and pepper on a flat tray, mix.

Pat dry the flounder using paper towels. Place the flounder fillets on the tray and press the flour on both sides, shake off the excess flour.

Place the oil in a frying pan and turn the heat to medium high. When the oil is hot add the flounder fillet cooking 3 minutes per side. Serve hot with lemon juice.

Baked Halibut and Kalamata Olives (serves 2)

- Two, 8-ounces of halibut fillet (16 ounces, total)
- salt, pepper or red pepper to taste
- 4 slices fresh lemon
- 2 Tbsp EVOO
- ½ cup kalamata olives
- ½ cup halved cherry tomatoes
- ½ cup fresh parsley, chopped
- 1 garlic clove, minced
- parchment paper

Place the halibut on a large parchment paper, rub salt and pepper. Add lemon slices on top of the fish. Sprinkle olive oil. Place olives, tomatoes, parsley, and garlic on top of the fish and around.

Close the fish in parchment paper and bake it at 350° F. in a preheated oven for 15 minutes. Serve.

Grilled Salmon (serves 2)

- Two, 4-ounce salmon steaks
- Salmoriglio sauce (see recipe)

Preheat the grill (stove top grill or barbecue grill, no more than medium high). Place the fish skin down and grill for 6-8 minutes. Flip once and cook for 2 minutes. Serve hot with 1 Tbsp of Salmoriglio sauce. Serve.

Baked Wild Salmon with Honey Mustard (serves 2)

- parchment paper
- Two, 8-ounce salmon steaks or one, 16-ounce salmon fillet
- salt and pepper to taste
- 1 Tbsp of honey mustard
- 1 Tbsp EVOO

Place the salmon onto parchment paper.
Rub the salmon with salt and pepper.
Rub the salmon with honey mustard. Drizzle olive oil over the salmon.
Bake in a 350° F. preheated oven for 12 to 15 minutes. Serve.

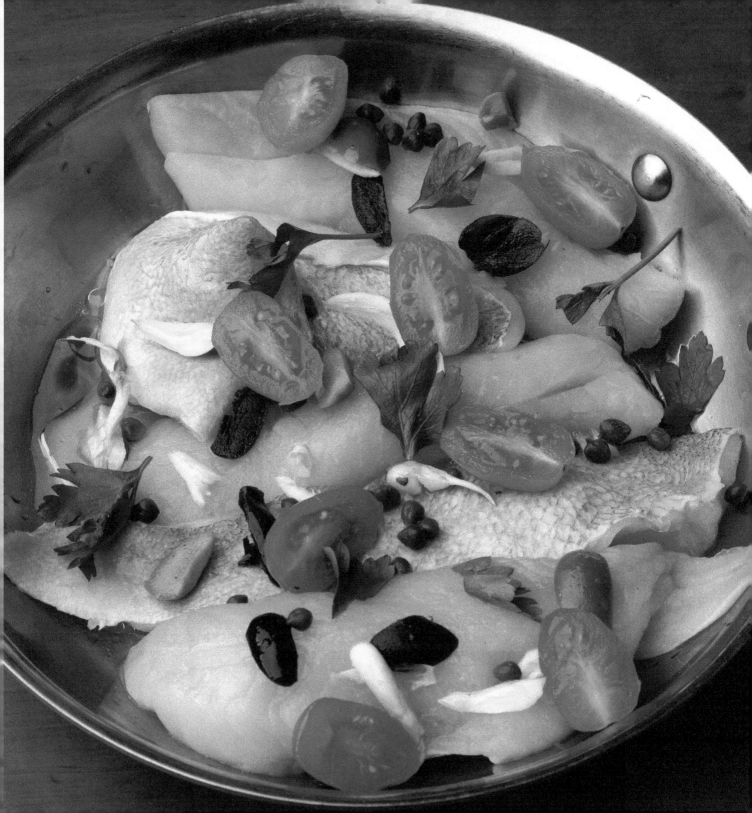

Grouper with Capers and Kalamata Olives (serves 2)
(snapper or halibut can be substituted)

- 1 fresh bread slice
- 1 fresh bread slice
- 1 garlic clove
- 1 small tomato
- 2 pitted kalamata olives
- 1 tsp capers
- ⅓ cup fresh parsley
- 1 Tbsp EVOO
- salt and pepper to taste
- 12 ounces grouper fillet

Remove the crust from the bread and place it in a food processor to obtain fresh bread crumbs. Add all the ingredients but the fish in the food processor and blend to a coarse paste.

Place the paste over the fish and bake in a 325° F. preheated oven for 10 minutes. Then turn and broil for 5 minutes. Serve hot.

Grilled Shrimp (serves 2)

- **8 medium-size shrimp**
- **1 Tbsp EVOO**
- **salt and pepper to taste**
- **1 garlic glove, minced**
- **juice from ⅛ lemon**
- **⅛ cup fresh parsley**

Place the cleaned shrimps in a bowl. Combine the other ingredients as the marinade in a separate bowl. Coat the shrimp generously with the marinade. Cover with plastic wrap for 2 to 4 hours. Place the shrimp over a hot stove top grill or barbecue. The shrimps are ready when they turn pink outside and they are white inside. Serve hot.

Sicilian Tuna in Agrodolce (sweet and sour sauce) (serves 2)

- 2 large Vidalia onions very thinly sliced
- 1 Tbsp EVOO
- salt and pepper to taste
- 4 Tbsp wine vinegar
- 1 Tbsp unrefined sugar
- tuna (8 ounces)

Turn the heat to low and cook the onions in olive oil in a covered pan. Add a couple of tablespoons of water. Cook until the onions are very soft. Add salt and pepper. Turn the heat to high and add the vinegar and sugar. Cook for 4 minutes stirring often.

Grill the tuna and add it to the onions. Serve hot.

Chicken

Baked Cornish Game Hen (serves 2)

- 1 Cornish hen
- ⅓ lemon juice from organic lemon
- 1 Tbsp EVOO
- salt and pepper to taste
- chopped sage, rosemary, thyme

With a scissor or a sharp knife cut the chest bone of the chicken and flatten the chicken.

Whisk lemon, EVOO, salt, pepper and herbs. Then rub it over the chicken cavity and skin.

Bake it at 400° F. for 15 minutes in a preheated oven, then turn the oven down to 350° F. and bake for 30 minutes. Serve.

Baked Chicken or Beef Cutlets (serves 2)

- 1 cup bread crumbs
- 1 Tbsp EVOO
- 1 Tbsp pecorino or Parmesan cheese
- ¼ cup chopped fresh parsley
- salt and pepper to taste
- 3.5 ounces thin chicken breast or thinly cut beef

Place the bread crumbs, EVOO, cheese, parsley, salt and pepper in a bowl and mix with your hands. Then cover the meat—both sides—with the bread mix. Bake at 350° F. in a preheated oven for 15 minutes. Serve.

Marinated Grilled, Free-Range Chicken (serves 2)

- Two, 3-ounce chicken breasts or boneless thighs
- parchment paper
- 2 Tbsp EVOO
- juice from ⅛ lemon
- salt and pepper to taste
- 2 garlic gloves, minced
- 2 tsp fresh or dry oregano

Place the meat between two parchment papers and pound to a thinner even steak. Mix the marinade in a bowl with EVOO, lemon juice, salt, pepper, garlic, and oregano.

Place the pounded meat into the bowl and coat it generously; then cover with plastic and place in the refrigerator from 2 to 4 hours.

Place the meat onto a hot grill, stove top or barbecue, and grill 2 to 3 minutes per side. Serve.

Free-Range Chicken Cacciatore (serves 2)

- 1 small onion, diced
- 1 carrot, diced
- 2 celery stalks, diced
- 1 Tbsp EVOO
- ⅓ cup chopped kalamata olives
- 2 tomatoes, diced
- Two, 3-ounce chicken breasts or boneless thighs
- salt, pepper or red pepper to taste

In a medium-size pan or Dutch oven over the stove, medium heat, sauté onion, carrot, celery, and EVOO until lightly brown.

Add olives and sauté for 2 minutes, add tomatoes.

Add chicken and cook for 20 minute with lid on. If the sauce is watery, remove the chicken and place on a dish. Let the sauce thicken at high heat for a few minutes, then add the chicken back and serve hot.

Beef

Marinated Grilled Pork Chops (serves 2)

- 1 Tbsp EVOO
- 1 Tbsp freshly squeezed lemon juice
- 1 tsp oregano
- salt and pepper to taste
- Two, 3-ounce pork chops

Prepare the marinade of EVOO, lemon, oregano, salt, and pepper. Place the meat into the marinade. Coat the meat generously.

Refrigerate for 2 to 4 hours.

Cook over a hot grill, medium-high stove top, or barbecue for 4 minutes, flip and cook for 3 minutes. Serve hot.

Marinated Grilled Sirloin (serves 2)

- Two, 3-ounce sirloin fillets
- 1 Tbsp EVOO
- 1 Tbsp fresh lemon juice
- 1 tsp oregano
- salt and pepper to taste

Combine EVOO, lemon juice, oregano, salt and pepper in a shallow bowl. Add the fillets coating the meat thoroughly. Marinate the fillets in the refrigerator for 3 to 6 hours. When ready to cook, turn the grill or stove-top-grill to high. Grill the meat for 5 to 6 minutes per side. Serve hot.

ENDNOTES

[2] ScienceDaily.ScienceDaily,2February2018.<www.sciencedaily.comreleases/2018/02/180202123836.htm>.)

[3] (The American Journal of Clinical Nutrition, 2017; 106 (4): 1041 DOI: 10.3945/%u200Bajcn.117.153635)

[4] (Association between Dietary Phenolic Acids and Hypertension in a Mediterranean Cohort, Nutrients, Vol 9, Issue 10, published online. DOI: 10.3390/nu9101069)

[5] (Rush University Medical Center. "MIND diet may slow cognitive decline in stroke survivors." ScienceDaily. ScienceDaily, 26 January 2018. <www.sciencedaily.com/releases/2018/01/180126110206.htm>.

[5] ScienceDaily. ScienceDaily, 15 January 2018. <www.sciencedaily.com/releases/2018/01/180115120542.htm>.)

[6] (Genome-wide meta-analysis associates HLA-DQA1/DRB1 and LPA and lifestyle factors with human longevity. Nature Communications, 2017; 8 (1) DOI: 10.1038/s41467-017-00934-5)

[7] (The Lancet).

[8] (Red and processed meat consumption and breast cancer: UK Biobank cohort study and meta analysis. Eur J Cancer. 2017;90:73-82.)

[9] (Mediterranean Dietary Pattern is Associated with Low Risk of Aggressive Prostate Cancer: MCC-Spain Study. The Journal of Urology, 2018; 199 (2): 430 DOI: 10.1016/j.juro.2017.08.087)

[10] (J Am Coll Cardiol. 1993 Aug;22(2):459-67.

[11] (Phylloquinone Intake Is Associated with Cardiac Structure and Function in Adolescents. The Journal of Nutrition, 2017; jn253666 DOI: 10.3945/jn.117.253666)

[12] (Bidirectional associations between psychosocial well-being and adherence to healthy dietary guidelines in European children: prospective findings from the IDEFICS study. BMC Public Health, 2017; 17 (1) DOI: 10.1186/s12889-017-4920-5)

[13] (Source Reference: Donin AS, et al. "Takeaway meal consumption and risk markers for coronary heart disease, type 2 diabetes and obesity in children aged 9-10 years: A cross-sectional study" Arch Dis Child 2017; DOI: 10.1136/archdischild-2017-312981.)

[14] (Transient triglyceridemia decreases vascular reactivity in young, healthy men without risk factors for coronary heart disease. Circulation. 1997 Nov 18;96(10):3266-8.)

[15] (Diabetes Care. 2006 Oct;29(10):2313-5. A high-carbohydrate, high-fiber meal improves endothelial function in adults with the metabolic syndrome.)

[16] (Adherence to Mediterranean Diet Reduces Incident Frailty Risk: Systematic Review and Meta-Analysis. Journal of the American Geriatrics Society, 2018; DOI: 10.1111/jgs.15251)

[17] (Journal of the Norwegian Medical Association 2011; 131 (5): 440 DOI: 10.4045/tidsskr.11.0081)

[18] (Cell Metab. 2014 Mar 4;19(3):407-17. doi: 10.1016/j.cmet.2014.02.006.

[19] Levine ME1, Suarez JA2, Brandhorst S2, Balasubramanian P2, Cheng CW2, Madia F3, Fontana L4, Mirisola MG5, Guevara-Aguirre J6, Wan J2, Passarino G7, Kennedy BK8, Wei M2, Cohen P2, Crimmins EM1, Longo VD9.)

[20] (USDA Agriculture Fact Book)

[21] Professor David Haslam, of the National Obesity Forum, stated: "The assumption has been made that increased fat in the bloodstream is caused by increased saturated fat in the diet. Modern scientific evidence is proving that refined carbohydrates and sugar in particular are actually the culprits."

[22] (PURE Trial - Lancet, Sept 11, 2018)

[23] These are the AHA 2017 statistics:

Rates of Heart Disease, Stroke and other Cardiovascular Diseases

• Deaths in the US. That's about 1 of every 3 deaths in the US.

• About 2,200 Americans die of cardiovascular disease each day, an average of 1 death every 40 seconds.

• Cardiovascular diseases claim more lives each year than all forms of cancer and Chronic Lower Respiratory Disease combined.

• About 92.1 million American adults are living with some form of cardiovascular disease or the after-effects of stroke. Direct and indirect costs of cardiovascular diseases and stroke are estimated to total more than $316 billion; that includes both health expenditures and lost productivity.

• Nearly half of all black adults have some form of cardiovascular disease, 47.7 percent of females and 46.0 percent of males. Food and Drug Administration (FDA)

[24] Juskevich JC, Guyer CG (August 1990). "Bovine growth hormone: human food safety evaluation". Science 249 (4971): 875-84. doi:10.1126/science.2203142. PMID 2203142 http://ec.europa.eu/food/fs/sc/scv/out19 en.html 1999 report of the European Commission Scientific Committee on Veterinary Measures relating to Public Health

[25] Myllys V, Honkanen-Buzalski T, Huovinen P, Sandholm M, Nurmi E (1994). "Association of changes in the bacterial ecology of bovine mastitis with changes in the use of milking machines and antibacterial drugs". Acta Vet Scand 35 (4): 363-9. PMID 7676918.

[26] (Sylvain Baughan J. 2002. What's under the coat of section 175.300? Available from: http://www.khlaw.com/showpublication.aspx?Show=2293 [accessed March 22, 2013].)

[27] [Comprehensive Reviews in Food Science and Food Safety. Vol 12. Issue 4, pages 439-453, July 2013]

[28] (Data Gaps in toxicity testing of chemicals allowed in food in the United States. Reproductive Toxicology 42(2013) 85-94)

[29] Toxicology Science 2006 Mar;90(91):178-87.

[30] Journal of Nutritional Science and Vitaminology 2000 Vol. 46 No. 3 pp. 130-136.

[31] Journal of Food Science Vol 41, Issue 4, pp. 949-951, July 1976.

[32] Toxic Effects of the Easily Avoidable Phthalates and Parabens. Altern Med Review. 2010 Sep; 15(3): 190-6)

[33] Dr. Walter Willet (intake of trans fatty acids and risk of coronary artery disease among women — Lancet. 1993 Mar 6;34 (8845): 581-5 showed that trans-fat increases the risk of heart disease.

[34] In 1975 Dr. Benjamin Feingold, "Why Your Child is Hyperactive" re: food dyes.

[35] ("Free Speech and Dietary Supplements" by Representative Ron Paul, Before the US House of Representatives, November 10, 2005)

[36] (American Heart Association. Circulation. 2011;123:933-44. Epub 2011 Jan 24).

[37] (JAMA, April 21, 1999—Vol 281, No. 15) (Percutaneous coronary intervention instable angina (ORBITA): a double-blind, randomized controlled trial. The Lance. Published: 02 November 2017)

[38] (Bodai BI, Nakata TE, Wong, WT, et al. Lifestyle medicine: a brief review of its dramatic impact on health and survival. PermJ. 2018;22:17-25.)

[39] (JAMA. 2011;305(1):43-49).

[40] "Anthony Samsel and Stephanie Seneff, "Glyphosate's Suppression of Cytochrome P450 Enzymes and Amino Acid Biosynthesis by the Gut Microbiome: Pathways to Modern Diseases" Entropy 2013, 15(4), 1416-1463; doi:10.3390/e15041416 (Download)

Robert M. Davidson, Ann Lauritzen and Stephanie Seneff, "Biological Water Dynamics and Entropy: A Biophysical Origin of Cancer and Other Diseases" Entropy 2013, 15, 3822-3876; doi:10.3390/e15093822 (Download)

Stephanie Seneff, Ann Lauritzen, Robert Davidson and Laurie Lentz-Marino, "Is Encephalopathy a Mechanism to Renew Sulfate in Autism?" Entropy 2013, 15, 372-406; doi:10.3390/e15010372 (Download)

Stephanie Seneff, Ann Lauritzen, Robert Davidson and Laurie Lentz-Marino, "Is Endothelial Nitric Oxide Synthase a Moonlighting Protein Whose Day Job is Cholesterol Sulfate Synthesis? Implications for Cholesterol Transport, Diabetes and Cardiovascular Disease." Entropy 2012, 14, 2492-2530; doi:10.3390/e14122492 (Download)

Stephanie Seneff, Robert M. Davidson and Jingjing Liu, "Is Cholesterol Sulfate Deficiency a Common Factor in Preeclampsia,

Autism, and Pernicious Anemia?" Entropy 2012, 14, 2265-2290; doi:10.3390/e14112265 (Download)

Samantha Hartzell and Stephanie Seneff, "Impaired Sulfate Metabolism and Epigenetics: Is There a Link in Autism?" Entropy 2012, 14, 1953-1977; doi:10.3390/e14101953 (Download)

Stephanie Seneff, Robert M. Davidson, and Jingjing Liu, "Empirical Data Confirm Autism Symptoms Related to Aluminum and Acetaminophen Exposure," Entropy 2012, 14, 2227-2253; doi:10.3390/e14112227 (Download)

Robert M. Davidson, and Stephanie Seneff, "The Initial Common Pathway of Inflammation, Disease, and Sudden Death," Entropy 2012, 14, 1399-1442; doi:10.3390/e14081399 (Download)

Stephanie Seneff, Glyn Wainwright, and Luca Mascitelli, "Nutrition and Alzheimer's Disease: The Detrimental Role of a High Carbohydrate Diet," European Journal of Internal Medicine 22 (2011) 134-140; doi:10.1016/j.ejim.2010.12.017 (Download)

Stephanie Seneff, Glyn Wainwright, and Luca Mascitelli, "Is the Metabolic Syndrome Caused by a High Fructose, and Relatively Low Fat, Low Cholesterol Diet?" Archives of Medical Science, 2011; 7, 1: 8-20; doi:10.5114/aoms.2011.20598 (Download)

See more at: http://naturalsociety.com/dr-stephanie-seneff-mit-scientist-explains-synergistic-effect-aluminum-glyphosate-poisoning-cause-skyrocketing-autism/#sthash.wCqjyA9p.dpuf

[41] 66. (Duffey KJ, et al. Food price and diet and health outcomes: 20 years of the CARDIA Study. Arch Intern Med. 2010; 170:420-6.)

[42] (WHO technical report series 916. Diet, nutrition and the prevention of excess weight gain and obesity. Report of a joint WHO/FAO expert consultation. Geneva: WHO, 2003.)

[43] (JAMA. 2002;288(14):1723-1727. doi:10.1001/jama.288.14.1723.)

[44 (JAMA. 2002;288(14):1728-1732. doi:10.1001/jama.288.14.1728.)

[45] BMJ 1997;314:1545-9.)

[46] (Bray GA, Nielsen SJ, Popkin BM. Consumption of high-fructose corn syrup in beverages may play a role in the epidemic of obesity. Am J Clin Nutr 2004;79:537-43.)

[47] (Nestle M Food Politics: How the Food Industry Influences Nutrition and Health. Berkeley University of California Press 2002)

[48] (Obes Res. 1999 Nov;7(6):564-71.) (Int J Obes Relat Metab Disord. 2000 Oct;24(10):1353-9.)

[49] (Public Health Nutrition / Volume 17 / Issue 11 / November 2014, pp 2445-2452)

[50] (Child Obes. 2012 Jun;8(3):251-4. doi: 10.1089/chi.2012.0016.)

[51] (Bowman SA, Gortmaker SL, Ebbeling CB, Pereira MA, Ludwig DS. Effects of fast-food consumption on energy intake and diet quality among children in a national household survey. Pediatrics 2004;113:112-8.)

[52] (Prev Med. 2001 Apr;32(4):303-10.)

[53] (J Nutr Educ Behav. 2014 Jan;46(1):75-81. doi: 10.1016/j.jneb.2013.10.008.)

[54] (Am J Prev Med. 2007 May;32(5):383-8.)

[55] Physicians Health Study - J Hypertens. 2008 Feb;26(2):215-22)

[56] (S. Sultan and N. Hynes, "The Ugly Side of Statins. Systemic Appraisal of the Contemporary Un Known Unknowns," Open Journal of Endocrine and Metabolic Diseases, Vol. 3 No. 3, 2013, pp. 179-185. doi:10.4236/ojemd.2013.33025.)

[58] [Jama 2000;283(3):373-380]

[59] [BMJ. 2012;344:d7373]

[60] (Spatial organization of a model 15-member human gut microbiota established in gnotobiotic mice. Proceedings of the National Academy of Sciences, 2017 DOI: 10.1073/ pnas.171596114)

61. (The Gut Microbiota of Healthy Aged Chinese Is Similar to That of the Healthy Young. mSphere, 2017; 2 (5): e00327-17 DOI: 10.1128/mSphere.00327-17)

[61a] (Clinical/Narrative Review

Subject Category: Clinical/Narrative Review

Citation: Clinical and Translational Gastroenterology (2015) 6, e91; doi:10.1038/ctg.2015.16 Published online 18 June 2015

The Influence of the Gut Microbiome on Obesity, Metabolic Syndrome and Gastrointestinal Disease OPEN

Parth J Parekh1, Luis A Balart1 and David A Johnson2

1Department of Internal Medicine, Division of Gastroenterology and Hepatology, Tulane University, New Orleans, Louisiana, USA

2Department of Internal Medicine, Division of Gastroenterology and Hepatology, Eastern Virginia Medical School, Norfolk, Virginia, USA

Correspondence: DA Johnson, M.D., MACG, FASGE, Department of Internal Medicine, Division of Gastroenterology and Hepatology, Eastern Virginia Medical School, Norfolk, Virginia 23510, USA. E-mail: dajevms@aol.com

Received 29 December 2014; Accepted 13 April 2015

Top of page

Abstract

[62] (Science 06 Sep 2013: Vol. 341, Issue 6150, DOI: 10.1126/science.1241214)

[63] (Nature. 2012 Aug 30;488(7413):621-6. doi: 10.1038/nature11400. Cho I1, Yamanishi S, Cox L, Methe BA, Zavadil J, Li K, Gao Z, Mahana D, Raju K, Teitler I, Li H, Alekseyenko AV, Blaser MJ.

[64] (Science, Vol. 357, Issue 6354, pp. 912-916, DOI: 10.1126/science.aan0677

[65] (Cell Host & Microbe, 2017; DOI: 10.1016/j.chom.2017.11.004 *Cell Host &Microbe*, 2017; DOI: 10.1016/j.chom.2017.11.003)

[66] (Fiber-Mediated Nourishment of Gut Microbiota Protects against Diet-Induced Obesity by Restoring IL-22-Mediated Colonic Health. Cell Host & Microbe, 2018; 23 (1):

[67] (Benefits of polyphenols on gut microbiota and implications in human health, The Journal of Nutritional Biochemistry, published online, DOI: 10.1016/j.jnutbio.2013.05.001)

[68] (Int J Food Microbiol. 2004 Jan 1;90(1):9-14.)

[69] (Dietary broccoli impacts microbial community structure and attenuates chemically induced colitis in mice in an Ah receptor dependent manner. Journal of Functional Foods, 2017; 37: 685 DOI: 10.1016/j.jff.2017.08.038)

[70] (Brain, Behavior, and Immunity, 2011; 25 (3): 397 DOI: 10.1016/j.bbi.2010.10.023)

[71] (Microbiome20175:102 https://doi.org/10.1186/s40168-017-0321-3

[80] (Pharmacy & Therapeutics. 2015 Apr; 40(4): 277—283.)

[81] (Nutrients. 2014 Nov; 6(11): 4822-4838.)

[82] (Effect of the Apolipoprotein E Genotype on Cognitive Change During a Multidomain Lifestyle Intervention. JAMA Neurology, 2018;)

[83] (Ornish. Proc Nat Acad Sci USA 2008; 105:8369)

[84] (Ornish, Lancet Oncol. 2013; 14(11): 1112-20

Fernandez, Elizabeth (2013-09-16). "Lifestyle Changes May Lengthen Telomeres, A Measure of Cell Aging". http://www.ucsf.edu/. University of California, San Francisco)

[85] Experimental Gerontology (November 2013), 1266-73

[86] (Clin Invest Med. 2006 Jun;29(3):154-8.

The Mediterranean diet in secondary prevention of coronary heart disease. de Lorgeril M1, Salen P.)

[87] Michael Fenech, CSIRO Genome Health and Nutrigenomics Laboratory

[88] (Neural Plasticity, Vol 2014, Article ID 563160)

[89] (Neuroscience. 2008 Aug 26; 155(3): 751-759)

[90] (Nature Communications 5, Article Number: 3746 (2014)

[91] (Environ Health Perspect. 2007 Dec; 115(12): A582-A589.)

[92] (British Journal of Nutrition, 2015; 1 DOI: 10.1017/S0007114515002093).

[93] (Tabung FK, Liu L, Wang W, et al. Association of dietary inflammatory potential with colorectal cancer risk in men and women. JAMA Oncol. Published online January 1)

[94] (Nature, 2017; 552 (7685): 355 DOI: 10.1038/nature25158)

[95] (Mechanistic Links Underlying the Impact of C-Reactive Protein on Muscle Mass in Elderly. Cellular Physiology and Biochemistry, 2017; 267 DOI: 10.1159/000484679)\

[96] (Rubin Naiman. Dreamless: the silent epidemic of REM sleep loss. Annals of the New York Academy of Sciences, 2017; DOI: 10.1111/nyas.13447)

[97] (Arch Gerontol Geriatr. 1996;22 Suppl 1:419-22.

Aspects of sleep in centenarians.

Spadafora FL1, Curti A, Teti R, Belmonte M, Castagna A, Mercurio M, Infusino P, Tavernese G, Iannazzo PS, Iorio C, Mattace R.)

[98] (Arch Intern Med. 2007 Feb 12;167(3):296-301.

Siesta in healthy adults and coronary mortality in the general population.

Naska A1, Oikonomou E, Trichopoulou A, Psaltopoulou T, Trichopoulos D.)

An interesting study performed at Harvard Medical School showed that napping improves cognitive function.

[99] (Nature Neuroscience 5, 677 - 681 (2002)

Published online: 28 May 2002; | doi:10.1038/nn864

The restorative effect of naps on perceptual deterioration

Sara C. Mednick1, Ken Nakayama1, Jose L. Cantero2, Mercedes Atienza2, Alicia A. Levin2, Neha Pathak2 & Robert Stickgold2)

[100] (Nature Neuroscience 10, 385 - 392 (2007)

Published online: 11 February 2007 | doi:10.1038/nn1851

A deficit in the ability to form new human memories without sleep

Seung-SchikYoo 1, Peter T Hu2, Ninad Gujar2, Ferenc A Jolesz1 & Matthew P Walker2)

[101] American Journal of Clinical Nutrition, 2018 DOI: 10.1093/ajcn/nqx030)

[102] (Swati Chopra, Aman Rathore, Haris Younas, Luu V. Pham, Chenjuan Gu, Aleksandra Beselman, Il-Young Kim, Robert R. Wolfe, Jamie Perin, VsevolodY. Polotsky, Jonathan C. Jun. Obstructive Sleep Apnea Dynamically Increases Nocturnal Plasma Free Fatty Acids, Glucose, and Cortisol during Sleep. The Journal of Clinical Endocrinology & Metabolism, 2017; DOI: 10.1210/ jc.2017-00619)

[103] http://www.reynoldsriskscore.org

[104] http://www.cvriskcalculator.com/

[105] https://www.framinghamheartstudy.org/risk-functions/cardiovascular-disease/10-year-risk. php#

[106] https://www.nhlbi.nih.gov/health/educational/lose_wt/BMI/bmicalc.htm.

[107] The American Heart Association, heart.org.

[108] (Source Reference: Lean M, et al. "Primary care-led weight management for remission of type 2 diabetes (DiRECT): an open-label, cluster-randomized trial" Lancet 2017; DOI:10.1016/ S0140-6736(17)33102-1.)

[109] (N Engl j Med 2013; 368:1279-1290 April 4, 2013DOI: 10.1056/NEJMoa1200303)

[110] (BMC Medicine, 2013).

[111] (Olive component oleuropein promotes -cell insulin secretion and protects -cells from amylin amyloid induced cytotoxicity. Biochemistry, 2017; DOI: 10.1021/acs.biochem.7b00199)

[112] JAMA Intern Med. 2015;175(11):1752-1760

[113] (Ophthalmology. 2016 Nov 5. pii: S0161-6420(16)31351-3. doi: 10.1016/j. ophtha.2016.09.019.) researchers discovered that this anti-inflammatory diet has a protective effect for the development of AMD.

[114] The Lyon Diet Heart Study (Circulation, 1999).

[115] JAMA in 2004

[116] (NEJM, 2008).

[117] Published online July 17, 2017. doi:10.1111/dom.13060.)

[118] (The Journals of Gerontology: Series A, 2018; 73 (1): 1 DOI: 10.1093/gerona/glx212)

[119] CRY2 and FBXL3 Cooperatively Degrade c-MYC. Molecular Cell, 2016; DO10.1016/j. molcel.2016.10.012).

[120] (FASEB J. 2016 Sep;30(9):3117-23. doi: 10.1096/fj.201600269RR. Epub 2016 Jun 2).

[121] (Physiol Behav. 2014 Jul;134:44-50. doi: 10.1016/j.physbeh.2014.01.001. Epub 2014 Jan 24.)

[122] (Am J Clin Nutr January 2014 vol. 99 no. 1 181-197).

[123] (Ann Neurol. 2013 Oct;74(4):580-91. doi: 10.1002/ana.23944. Epub 2013 Sep 16.)

[124] (BMC Med. 2015; 13: 215.)

[125] (Source Reference: Morris MC, et al. "Nutrients and bioactives in green leafy vegetables and cognitive decline - Prospective study" Neurology 2018;90:1-9; DOI:10.1212/ WNL.0000000000004815.)

[127] (Am J Clin Nutr. 2012 Apr;95(4):818-24. doi: 10.3945/ajcn.111.027383. Epub 2012 Feb 22.)

[128] (Scientific Reports, 2017; 7 (1) DOI: 10.1038/s41598-017-17520-w)

[129] (Shukla AP, Andono J, Touhamy SH, et al. Carbohydrate-last meal pattern lowers postprandial glucose and insulin excursions in type 2 diabetes BMJ Open Diabetes Research and Care 2017;5:e000440. doi: 10.1136/bmjdrc-2017-000440)

[131] (JAMA. 1998;280(23):2001-2007. doi:10.1001/jama.280.23.2001)

[132] (*JAMA*. 1983;249(1):54-59. doi:10.1001/jama.1983.03330250034024)
(The Lancet , Volume 336 , Issue 8708 , 129 - 133)
(JAMA. 1998;280(23):2001-2007. doi:10.1001/jama.280.23.2001)

[133] (European Respiratory Journal, December 2017 DOI: 10.1183/13993003.02286-2016)

[134] (Atherosclerosis. 2006 Apr;185(2):438-45. Epub 2005 Aug 10.)

[135] (Clin Nutr. 2013 Apr;32(2):200-6. doi: 10.1016/j.clnu.2012.08.022. Epub 2012 Sep 3.)

[136] (Biol Res. 2004;37(2):209-15.)

[137] (Clin Nutr. 2013 Apr;32(2):200-6. doi: 10.1016/j.clnu.2012.08.022. Epub 2012 Sep 3.)

[138] (Br J Nutr. 2007 Oct;98 Suppl 1:S111-5.)

[139] (Drugs Exp Clin Res. 2003;29(5-6):235-42.)

[140] (The Journal of Experimental Medicine, 2017; jem.20161066 DOI: 10.1084/jem.20161066)

[141] (Beneficial effects of low alcohol exposure, but adverse effects of high alcohol intake on glymphatic function. Scientific Reports, 2018; 8)

[142] (Food and Nutrition Board, Institute of Medicine. Dietary Reference Intakes for Energy, Carbohydrate, Fiber, Fat, Fatty Acids, Cholesterol, Protein, and Amino Acids (Macronutrients). Washington, DC: National Academies Press; 2005.)

[143] (Threapleton DE, Greenwood DC, Evans CE, et al. Dietary fiber intake and risk of first stroke: a systematic review and meta-analysis. Stroke. 2013;44:1360-1368.)

[144] (Coffee consumption and health: umbrella review of meta-analyses of multiple health outcomes. BMJ, 2017)

[145] (PLOS. "Caffeine from four cups of coffee protects the heart with the help of mitochondria." Science-Daily. ScienceDaily, 21 June 2018. <www.sciencedaily.com/ releases/2018/06/180621141008. htm>.)

[146] (Stevens Institute of Technology. "The scent of coffee appears to boost performance in math: Smelling a coffee-like scent, which has no caffeine in it, creates an expectation for students that they will perform better on tests." ScienceDaily. ScienceDaily, 17 July 2018. <www. sciencedaily.com/ releases/2018/07/180717125836.htm>.)

[147] (Differences of energy expenditure while sitting versus standing: A systematic review and meta analysis.
European Journal of Preventive Cardiology, 2018; 204748731775218)

[148] (JAMA. 2003 Jul 9;290(2):215-21.)

[148] (JAMA Intern Med. 2015 Jun;175(6):959-67. doi: 10.1001/jamainternmed.2015.0533.)

[149] (Source Reference: Lachman S, et al. "Impact of physical activity on the risk of cardiovascular disease in middle-aged and older adults: EPIC Norfolk prospective population study" Eur J Prev Cardiol 2017; DOI: 10.1177/2047487317737628.)

[150] (Accelerometer-Measured Physical Activity and Mortality in Women Aged 63 to 99. Journal of the American Geriatrics Society, 2017; DOI: 10.1111/jgs.15201)

[151] (Changes in Daily Steps and Body Mass Index and Waist to Height Ratio during Four Year Follow-Up in Adults: Cardiovascular Risk in Young Finns Study. International Journal of Environmental Research and Public Health, 2017; 14 (9): 1015 DOI: 10.3390/ ijerph14091015)

[152] (JAMA Intern Med. 2015 Jun;175(6):970-7. doi: 10.1001/jamainternmed.2015.0541.)

[153] (The American Journal of Medicine , Volume 128 , Issue 11 , 1171 - 1177)

[154] (Body weight homeostat that regulates fat mass independently of leptin in rats and mice. Proceedings of the National Academy of Sciences, 2017; 201715687 DOI: 10.1073/ pnas.1715687114)

[155] (Epigenetics. 2014 Dec;9(12):1557-69. doi: 10.4161/15592294.2014.982445.)

[156] (Cell Metabolism , Volume 17 , Issue 2 , 162 - 184)

[157] (Rehfeld K, Muller P, Aye N, et al. Dancing or fitness sport? The effects of two training programs on hippocampal plasticity and balance abilities in healthy seniors. Front Hum Neurosci. 2017;11:305. doi: 10.3389/fnhum.2017.00305.)

[158] (Can Exercise Improve Cognitive Symptoms of Alzheimer's Disease? A Meta-Analysis. Journal of the American Geriatrics Society, 2018)

[159] (Arch Intern Med. 2001;161(14):1703-1708.)

[160] (Immunology and Cell Biology (2000) 78, 532—535)

[161] (Neuropsychologia, 2018; 108: 73 DOI: 10.1016/j.neuropsychologia.2017.11.029)

[162] (http://www.apa.org/research/action/fit.aspx).

[163] (JAMA. 2002 Nov 13;288(18):2300-6.)

[164] (Front Public Health. 2013; 1: 11.)

[165] (Environ Health Prev Med. 2000 Oct; 5(3): 85—89.) (NEJM Vol 338, Number 2, Page 94)

[166] (Malays J Med Sci. 2008 Oct; 15(4): 9-18.)

[167] (JAMA Intern Med. 2013;173(1):76-77.

[168] (Sheldon Cohen, Denise Janicki-Deverts, William J. Doyle, Gregory E. Miller, Ellen Frank, Bruce S. Rabin, and Ronald B. Turner. Chronic stress, glucocorticoid receptor resistance, inflammation, and disease risk. PNAS, April 2, 2012 DOI: 10.1073/pnas.1118355109).

[169] (JAMA, November 26, 2008 - Vol 300, No 20)

[170] (Okereke OI, Prescott J, Wong JYY, Han J, Rexrode KM, De Vivo I. High Phobic Anxiety Is Related to Lower Leukocyte Telomere Length in Women. Zhang XY, ed. PLoS ONE. 2012;7(7):e40516. doi:10.1371/journal.pone.0040516.)

[171] (Wolkowitz OM, Mellon SH, Epel ES, et al. Leukocyte Telomere Length in Major Depression: Correlations with Chronicity, Inflammation and Oxidative Stress - Preliminary Findings. Kiechl S, ed. PLoS ONE. 2011;6(3):e17837. doi:10.1371/journal.pone.0017837.)

[172] (Ranabir S, Reetu K. Stress and hormones. Indian Journal of Endocrinology and Metabolism. 2011;15(1):18-22. doi:10.4103/2230-8210.77573.)

[173] (Nat Rev Cardiol. 2012 Apr 3;9(6):360-70. doi: 10.1038/nrcardio.2012.45.)

[174] (Psychosom Med. 1980 Sep;42(5):493-7.)

[175] (Psychosom Med. 2006 Sep-Oct;68(5):692-7.)

[176] (Pizzorno J. Glutathione! Integrative Medicine: A Clinician's Journal. 2014;13(1):8-12.)

[177] (Sauna Bathing and Incident Hypertension: A Prospective Cohort Study. American Journal of Hypertension, 2017; DOI: 10.1093/ajh/hpx102)

[178] (Science. 1988 Jul 29;241(4865):540-5.)

[179] (Soc Sci Med. 2006 Oct;63(8):2204-17. Epub 2006 Jun 23.)

[180] (Psychosomatics. 2007 May-Jun;48(3):211-6

[181] (Int J Psychophysiol. 2006 Nov;62(2):328-36. Epub 2006 Aug 14.)

[182] (J Biosoc Sci. 2006 Nov;38(6):835-42. Epub 2006 Jan 27.)

[183] (Student perception of group dynamics predicts individual performance: Comfort and equity matter. PLOS ONE, 2017; 12 (7): e0181336 DOI: 10.1371/journal.pone.0181336)

[184] (Changes in marital quality over 6 years and its association with cardiovascular disease risk factors in men: findings from the ALSPAC prospective cohort study. Journal of Epidemiology and Community Health, 2017; jech-2017-209178 DOI: 10.1136/jech-2017-209178)

[185] (Medical Humanities, 2017; medhum-2017-011195 DOI: 10.1136/medhum-2017-011195)

[186] (Catherine Meads, Josephine Exley. A SYSTEMATIC REVIEW OF GROUP WALKING IN PHYSICALLY HEALTHY PEOPLE TO PROMOTE PHYSICAL ACTIVITY. International Journal of Technology Assessment in Health Care, 2018; 1)

ACKNOWLEDGMENTS

A book is a great example of a community effort. The community behind The Sicilian Secret Diet is quite large and extends over multiple continents and 5000 years of history. Our children, Francesca, who is a Doctoral candidate in Nurse Practice at Columbia University, with a background in psychology and nutrition, our son, Danny, who is a permaculture farmer in North Carolina, and our daughter-in-law, Teresa, who is a rural physician with a strong interest in nutrition and lifestyle medicine, are our most effective critics and have helped tremendously in the editing of the book. Our families, including our siblings, cousins, and nieces and nephews have always lovingly supported our work and we enjoyed together many family dinners where we ate The Sicilian Diet style food.

We would like to thank our dear friend, Keith Frankel, who is CEO and Founder of Vitaquest Intl, for his support and encouragement to write this book. Keith introduced us to Alan Morell, who is CEO of The Creative Management Agency, who is our agent and has worked tirelessly to see this project to completion.

I would also like to thank my partners, Scott Berliner RhP and Frank Lipman, M.D., in our advanced anti-aging practice in New York City, CorAeon. Scott is a compound pharmacist like no other, an expert in nutrition, supplements and hormones. Frank is an expert in detoxification diets, gut microbiome and cognition, and he has published 5 books and is about to publish 2 more on longevity and sleep.

Finally we would like to thank John Colby Jr., Publisher at Brick Tower Press and his incredible team and in particular Glen Edelstein for his excellent editing and design skills. And we would also like to thank Louie Papio, our photographer, who is a food photography artist.

ABOUT THE AUTHORS

Dr. Giovanni Campanile is a Harvard trained Cardiologist - Lahey Clinic Foundation, Massachusetts General Hospital, New England Deaconess Hospital. He was the cardiologist on-call for former President of the United States, George H.W. Bush.

Former director of the Dean Ornish Intensive Cardiac Rehabilitation Program and former director of Integrative Nutrition and Integrative Cardiology at the Chambers Center for Well Being at Morristown Medical Center / Atlantic Health System. Dr. Campanile has multiple board certifications in Internal Medicine, Cardiology, Interventional Cardiology, the American Board of Integrative and Holistic Medicine and The American Academy of Anti-Aging and Regenerative Medicine. He is Assistant Professor of Medicine at Rutgers New Jersey Medical School and has been an instructor for cardiologists in-training at Lenox Hill Hospital in NYC and Columbia University Mount Sinai, Miami.

Researcher at the world-renowned Framingham Heart Study, and recently investigated integrative modalities with the National Institutes of Health, Rutgers New Jersey Medical School, Duke University and Yale University. Co-edited and wrote the chapters on Sports Cardiology and Lifestyle Medicine for the first textbook on Iatrogenicity in Cardiovascular Medicine.

Dr. Campanile has written articles on nutrition for Shape and Men's Fitness Magazine.

Dr. Campanile has been practicing Clinical, Preventive, and Integrative Cardiology for over 15 years and has been a member of an advisory board at Bastyr University. He has been an instructor of nutrition, herbology and integrative medicine at Florida Atlantic University, and is a certified aromatherapist. Dr. Campanile has been named "Top Doctor" in cardiology by *New Jersey Monthly* magazine for multiple years.

Sandra Cammarata, M.D. was born in Milan, in northern Italy, but grew up in Catania, Sicily.

She graduated *Summa Cum Laude* from Catania Medical school and moved with her husband, Giovanni Campanile, to the United States where she specialized in General Psychiatry and Child and Adolescent Psychiatry at Tufts University.

Selected in 2020 as one of Castle Connolly's "Exceptional Women in Medicine,"Sandra has been practicing Psychiatry in private practice in New Jersey and has been awarded the Castle Connolly best New Jersey Child and Adolescent Psychiatrist award for multiple years. She successfully integrates nutrition and healthy eating in the treatment of her patients.

In 2013 she opened a gourmet ancient grain fresh pasta restaurant in Brooklyn, New York, using her family's traditional Sicilian recipes.

Her home is warmly open to friends and family in appreciation of the Sicilian diet.

CPSIA information can be obtained
at www.ICGtesting.com
Printed in the USA
BVHW050750111121
621189BV00004B/217